Sensual Sex

❖ ❖ ❖

Sensual Sex clearly illustrates for the reader the continuum from sensuality to desire to arousal. The exercises in the book have a unique focus on sensuality, and Beverly Engel takes careful note of the different stages couples go through in a relationship. The information on aromatherapy is especially appropriate in this book centering on opening up to all five senses. *Sensual Sex* also contains some of the best descriptions I've ever read of oral sex—one of the most sensual of pleasures.

> — Barbara Keesling, Ph.D.,
> author of *Sexual Pleasure, Sexual Healing,*
> *Making Love Better than Ever*

Sensual Sex is an informative, practical guide toward an all-encompassing sexuality. This clear and easy-to-read book will prove informative and rewarding, helping readers to harness all their senses and emotions.

> —Alan R. Hirsch, M.D.,
> author of *Scentsational Sex*

This book is dedicated to

Ed Djergian,

Bette Harrell,

and Barbara Roberts

May you rest in peace, love, and bliss

ORDERING

Trade bookstores in the U.S. and Canada please contact:

Publishers Group West
1700 Fourth Street, Berkeley CA 94710
Phone: (800) 788-3123   Fax: (510) 528-3444

Hunter House books are available at bulk discounts for textbook course adoptions; to qualifying community, healthcare, and government organizations; and for special promotions and fundraising. For details please contact:

Special Sales Department
Hunter House Inc., PO Box 2914, Alameda CA 94501-0914
Phone: (510) 865-5282 Fax: (510) 865-4295
e-mail: marketing@hunterhouse.com

Individuals can order our books from most bookstores or by calling toll free: (800) 266-5592

Sensual Sex

❖ ❖ ❖

*Arousing Your Senses and Deepening the Passion
in Your Relationship*

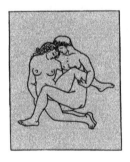

BEVERLY ENGEL, M.F.C.C.

Library of Congress Cataloging-in-Publication Data
Engel, Beverly.
    Sensual sex : awakening your senses and deepening the passion in your relationship / Beverly Engel. - 1st ed.
    p. cm.
    Includes bibliographical references.
    ISBN 0-89793-245-5

1. Sex instruction. 2. Sexual excitement. 3. Sense (Philosophy). 4. Intimacy (Psychology). I. Title
HQ31.E745 1999
613.9'6 - dc21   98-52742
                                              CIP

PROJECT CREDITS

Cover Design: Madeleine Budnick   *Book Design:* Brian Dittmar
Copy Editor: Mimi Kusch   *Project Editors:* Kiran Rana, Lisa Lee
Managing Editor: Wendy Low   *Editorial Assistant:* Jennifer Rader
Acquisitions Coordinator: Jeanne Brondino
Proofreader: Lee Rappold   *Indexer:* Kathy Talley-Jones
Publicity: Marisa Spatafore   *Marketing Intern:* Monique Portegies
Customer Support: Christina Sverdrup, Joel Irons
Order Fulfillment: A & A Quality Shipping Services
Publisher: Kiran S. Rana

Interior illustrations taken from *Maillol Erotic Woodcuts,*
Dover Publications, Mineola, NY: 1988.

9 8 7 6 5 4 3 2   First Edition   02 03

CONTENTS

Humans are tuned for relationship.

The eyes, the skin, the tongue, ears,

and nostrils—all are gates where our

body receives the nourishment of otherness.

— FROM *THE SPELL OF THE SENSUOUS* BY DAVID ABRAM

Acknowledgments

The author is grateful for permission to reprint the poetry selection on page 66 from *30 Songs of Dissolution* by Glenna Luschei, Cerrillos, NM: San Marcos Press, ©1977. Used by permission of the author.

This book is a compilation of many years of study and training. Although it is not possible to thank everyone who taught or influenced me, I wish to express my gratitude to some of the many experts I have learned from: William Hartman and Marilyn Fithian, Julia Heiman and Joseph LoPiccolo, Lonnie Barbach, Helen Singer Kaplan, John Money, and Masters and Johnson. I would also like to thank fellow members of the human potential movement: George Leonard, Bernard Gunther, and Len Harris; the many people I met through the years at Esalen and Elysium; and my friends from I.P.S.A.

I would like to acknowledge all those whose research or clinical experience added depth and authority to this book: Masters and Johnson, Ashley Montague, Lonnie Barbach, Dr. Patricia Love, Valerie Gennari Cooksley, Georg Feuerstein, Daniel Beaver, and David and Ellen Ramsdale.

A special tribute goes to Barbara Roberts, my dear friend who introduced me to I.P.S.A., to the Los Angeles Sex Information Helpline, and to the Society for the Scientific Study of Sex; Ed Djergian, who taught me to discover the sensuousness in all of nature; and Bette Harrell who taught me how to love.

Last, but not least, I wish to acknowledge those at Hunter House: Kiran Rana and Lisa Lee for their help in the development of the project, Mimi Kusch for her copy editing, Jennifer Rader, editorial assistant, Wendy Low, managing editor, and Marisa Spatafore, publicity director.

Introduction

Because of the threat of AIDS and the growing divorce rate, more and more couples are trying to stay together and to remain monogamous. They are hungry for advice on just how to do this, and books about how to "put the spark back" into relationships have been growing increasingly popular. Yet many of these books place too heavy an emphasis on the physical techniques of lovemaking. Although such books may be useful for learning about certain basic sexual techniques, they often overemphasize performance and orgasm, while ignoring the more profound feelings associated with sensual pleasures and intimate love. Thus, instead of helping to bring lovers closer together to create a mutual emotional refuge from the demands of everyday life, many current sex books frequently bring the performance pressures and anxieties of the working world into the bedroom.

Moreover, many of these books recommend activities that one or both partners may resist or resent. This is particularly true of books that require couples to engage in lengthy discussions about their sexual issues and desires or to experiment with sexual fantasies or role-playing. Because of our cultural training, most women are able to talk about their emotions better than men are. Conversely, because males are given more permission to be sexual in our culture, men tend to be more willing to experiment sexually than are women. Fortunately, both men and women will welcome the opportunity to reconnect with each other in the nonthreatening, physically pleasurable ways suggested in this book.

Sensual Sex will do what many of the popular couples books have promised but have often not delivered. It will offer couples techniques that will help them to reignite their passions, not by encouraging sexual fantasies, role-playing, or sexual experimentation but by helping them establish real intimacy and trust and by helping them to awaken the natural, spontaneous, exquisite pleasures of sensuality.

Although sensuality may not seem like a cutting-edge topic for a book of this type, I strongly believe that it is a subject whose time has come. As the expression goes, "everything old is new again," and that applies to tenderness, "slow-handed" touching, and taking the time to connect on an intimate level. Indeed, the old ways are reemerging, as we become nostalgic for a simpler, more predictable life. After years of striving for the much-lauded superorgasms, multiple orgasms, and simultaneous orgasms, we are finally coming back to the basics—sensuality, touch, and intimacy.

In the 1970s, during what was called the "human potential movement," massage, sensual touch, and sensuality training became increasingly popular as we switched our focus from materialism to more humane endeavors. Growth centers like Esalen and Kairos in California offered classes and workshops in subjects such as Esalen massage, meditation, and stress reduction. Instead of going out for an expensive dinner and the theater or the movies, couples frequently signed up for a course in sensuality training. Instead of redecorating the house, many spent their extra money on massage lessons or weekend workshops on learning how to achieve more intimacy. Even big business got into the act by paying for their employees to receive "sensitivity training," with its emphasis on reconnecting with one's senses, learning better communication skills, and becoming more sensitive to others' feelings.

Then came the eighties, and the pendulum swung in the opposite direction. Money was no longer considered the root of all evil. Expensive dinners, designer clothing, and beautiful homes were valued far more than tending to our stress levels, learning to communicate with our partners, or taking time to smell the roses. We no longer had time for such "touchy-feely" hogwash. Those who advocated health food, alternative medicine, or the benefits of massage, acupressure, or tantric sex were written off as airheads. We worked hard, partied hard, and shopped till we dropped. Most growth centers closed due to lack of business, and sensitivity training fell by the wayside.

Now as we approach the millennium, we find that we have come full circle. Once again we recognize the price we've paid for placing so much importance on money and material possessions. Once again we are recognizing the important role relationships play, or should play, in our lives. And as we become oversaturated with reading about and trying out every possible variation on sex and recognize how empty we still feel, we have once again begun to value sensuality, touch, and intimacy.

Those of us who were researching sexuality and sensuality during the human potential movement have known for years about the importance of touch to healthy sexuality, intimacy, physical and emotional healing, and our overall well-being. Now that more of the general public is finally putting its stamp of approval on information we've had all along, we have mixed feelings. Naturally, we feel elated that suddenly more people are interested in massage and sensuality, but at the same time we are experiencing déjà vu. Haven't we already gone through this? Doesn't everyone already know this stuff?

The truth is that although many people already know about the importance of sensual touch, many do not. A large part of the population—all the twenty- and thirty-year-olds who missed the sexual revolution, for example—has never been introduced to the benefits of sensual caressing, focusing on the senses, and sensuality in general. And for many others who were around for the revolution, it seems as if the lessons learned from the human potential movement have been all but forgotten.

Therefore, it is my pleasure and honor to share with you information that literally changed my life and that has changed the lives of many other people through the years, information that I believe to be as important as any medical breakthrough, information that can change your life as well.

Although some of the wisdom I will share hearkens back to discoveries about sex made in the seventies and eighties, much of it has been updated, such as in the area of sexual fantasy. In addition, I have included information and exercises that represent new breakthroughs in sensuality and sexuality as well as current research on the effects of touch on our overall health and on our sexuality.

Because so many people are touch deprived, because so many are plagued with sexual problems and sexual fears, and because so many couples grow apart and even divorce because of a lack of physical connectedness, I have made the study of sensuality and touch a major focus in my life.

Sensual Sex is a compilation of all the wisdom I have collected during my many years as a sex therapist and sex educator. I began my professional career as a sex therapist and marriage counselor back in the mid-seventies, but my interest in sexuality and sensuality began much earlier. Having been both touch deprived and sexually abused as a child, I had a special interest in nonsexual touching. After taking some courses in massage I learned first-hand the healing qualities of sensual touch. I then began to teach sensuality training at various growth centers throughout California.

I later worked with and was trained by sex researchers and therapists Hartman and Fithian, who were considered the Masters and Johnson of the West Coast. A key part of this training was learning the sensate focus exercises I present to you in this book.

Today I am internationally recognized as an expert in the fields of sexuality and abuse, having been a sex therapist, sex educator, marriage counselor, and workshop leader for over twenty-four years and the best-selling author of ten nonfiction books, many of which deal with sexual issues.

Although much of the information in this book was gleaned from my many years of clinical experience, it also represents my years of study in the fields of psychology, sexuality, marriage counseling, and communication skills. I have personally created many of the exercises in this book, and have used them successfully with my clients throughout the years. Some of the exercises are variations of those offered by other sources, such as those inspired by ancient traditions such as tantra yoga and tantric sex. A few were created in the sixties and seventies by well-known therapists and workshop leaders, and others were created by sex researchers such as Masters and Johnson and Hartman and Fithian. Whenever possible, I have given credit to the creators of the exercises, but in many cases I was unable to do so, since some of the originators are unknown. Therefore, any oversight should be considered unintentional and will be corrected in future editions of the book.

Part I

❖ ❖ ❖

Sensual Joy

The only sin passion can commit is to be joyless.

— DOROTHY SAYERS

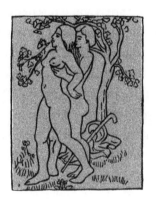

CHAPTER ONE

The Joys of
Sensual Sex

M ore than likely you are looking at or have purchased this book because you are searching for some answers. Perhaps you would like to know why your sex life isn't what you'd like it to be. Or perhaps you are looking for a way to regain the excitement you once felt with your partner. If you are a woman, perhaps you are having trouble becoming aroused or reaching orgasm, and if you are a man, you may be experiencing problems maintaining an erection or lasting as long as you'd like. Maybe you don't feel satisfied sexually, or fear you are not satisfying your partner. Or perhaps you are reading this book because you would like to have the kind of sex life that you imagine others are enjoying.

Although *Sensual Sex: Arousing Your Senses and Deepening the Passion in Your Relationship* can and will address all these concerns, you will find that they are not the focus of the book. Rather, we will focus more on awakening your senses than on your performance, more on helping you to sink into sensation rather than on your partner's pleasure, and perhaps most important, more on encouraging you to bask in the exquisite pleasure of touch than on expending your energy trying to reach orgasm. Only by doing these things will you be able to achieve the kind of sexual experiences that are your birthright, the kind of exquisitely sensual experiences of which we all dream.

As a marriage counselor and sex therapist, I have found that couples who suffer from sexual problems or a lack of sexual desire often don't need extensive therapy as much as they need to learn to refocus on sensual pleasure and sensual touch instead of on performance and orgasms.

Perhaps you are reading this book because you were attracted to the idea of sensual sex. You may already feel that your relationship could benefit from more touching, more tenderness, more sensuality. You may miss the way you and your partner used to touch each other when you were first together. The very words *sensual sex* may have been what attracted many of you to this book. These words may elicit fantasies of long, pleasurable evenings with your partner in a candlelit room with soft music playing, as you lose yourselves in each other's bodies.

Most men and women realize that they are capable of much more sexual pleasure and a much deeper relationship than they permit themselves to experience. They realize their relationships have room for growth in terms of sexual pleasure, playfulness, and intimacy. This is what *Sensual Sex: Arousing Your Senses and Deepening the Passion in Your Relationship* is all about: to encourage you to experience your partner on a deeper, more sensual, yet playful, level, to focus less on performance and orgasm and more on pleasure and surrender.

Sex is more than two bodies coming together to perform athletic acts. It is more than giving your partner an orgasm or getting one for yourself. Ideally, sex is a way for two people to connect on a deeper emotional level, to bask in the pleasure of each other's bodies, to linger over the sight, smell, taste, and touch of one another, to become lost in sensation.

Unfortunately, many of us have experienced a dulling of our senses brought on by our fast-paced lives. Our senses have become deadened by overstimulation and neglect. We are bombarded daily by a deafening array of sounds and an onslaught of smells. Our eyes are blinded by the harshness that surrounds us, and our bodies are squeezed into tiny compartments—everything from our compact cars to our cubicles at work. Our senses are so overstimulated that we automatically block out sensations in order to survive. And yet, at the same time, we are hungry for positive sensations—soothing sounds, satisfying tastes and smells, nature's beauty, and sensual and healing touch.

Most of us have become so hardened by daily stress that our bodies have lost the ability to relax into sensual joy, to become liquid with surrender. We've mastered the art of the "quickie," of the self-induced orgasm and of the mechanically aided orgasm. We've mastered the art of orgasms induced by fantasy and pornography, and yet we've lost the art of the slow, sensuous, spontaneous orgasm. We have become so sophisticated sexually that we now have books teaching us how to have all kinds of orgasms. Yet ironically, most of us are basically touch deprived. Finally, we've become so obsessed with physical perfection that we've stopped appreciating how much our other senses add to our sensual and sexual pleasure.

⑥ Beyond Performance and Orgasms ⑥

The premise of *Sensual Sex* is that by focusing more on pleasure than on performance, by slowing down and taking the time to connect more intimately, we can enjoy a deeply satisfying relationship with our partner that goes beyond orgasms, performance, and our striving for perfection. By becoming more attuned to all our senses, especially our sense of touch, we can develop an increasingly erotic relationship with both our own and our partner's body.

Through a series of innovative touching and sensuality exercises, *Sensual Sex* will help you to reconnect with and awaken to your body's exquisite pleasures, to luxuriate in your senses, to drink in delicious sensations. Each chapter of the book will encourage you to explore and experiment with different textures, sights, tastes, smells, and sounds. In addition, it will teach you caressing techniques that will encourage you to slow down, to focus all your attention on the point of contact between your body and your partner's, and to give up control and concern about performance. Finally, *Sensual Sex* will suggest ways for you to nurture your relationship on a daily basis, to both strengthen it and to imbue it with new energy and excitement.

Sensual Sex will help couples bend and curve into each other, to soften their hearts and surrender their senses. By helping you to reconnect with and appreciate both your own and your partner's body, it will help to alleviate many of your concerns about your body image. It will help you to discover new, exquisitely delightful sensations and to reach new heights of ecstasy together.

This book will also help you connect with the soul of your sensual and sexual relationship. As Thomas Moore stated in his book *Care of the Soul,* the great malady of the twentieth century is "loss of soul." We have grown empty and cold through our preoccupation with money, achievement, and excitement. *Soul* encompasses our profound experiences—deep connections with others, love, music, good food, and nature—that stay in our memories and touch us. These experiences fill our empty spots and warm our hearts. And a great deal of soul can be found in relationships that are sensuously intimate.

⑥ Sensual Sex ⑥

What is Sensual Sex? And how is it different from "ordinary" sex? Obviously, it is sex that is sensuous. But isn't all sex sensuous? The answer is both yes and no. By definition, the word sensuous means "relating to or consisting of the gratification of the senses or the indulgence of appetite." Sadly, most sex does not fulfill either of these needs. Sensual Sex, on the other hand, is deeply gratifying, primarily because it meets our deep hunger to connect with all our senses.

An integral part of learning to be more sensual, then, is to begin to focus on your senses of touch, smell, sight, taste, and hearing. By focusing in this way, you can intensify your sexual experiences and make them all the more delicious and joyful.

But Sensual Sex involves more than connecting with all our senses. Unlike ordinary sex, Sensual Sex is not goal oriented. There is no push for orgasm. Sensual Sex is relaxed and slow, more like a lazy river than a tumultuous ocean. Passion is present, but it is the kind of passion that builds up slowly, gaining momentum with time. Unlike the full-steam-ahead, get-there-as-fast-as-you-can mentality that so rules our culture, Sensual Sex is more like a slow burn—the water still reaches the boiling point, but it takes much longer to get there.

Sensual Sex is far more fulfilling, far more intimate than routine sex. By involving all the senses, by taking the time to really take in and enjoy your partner's body, you will satisfy not only your desire for an orgasm but also your desire for your partner and for intimacy.

Sensual Sex is flowing, spontaneous, exploratory. Instead of following the same mundane routine, you allow the next feeling and touch to unfold. One moment you may feel playful, the next reverent.

Sensual Sex is creative and playful. It encourages you to allow your spontaneity and imagination to take over so you can discover new sensations and new joys. Once you lose your compulsive need to give and receive an orgasm, you begin to reconnect with the more joyous side of sex. You learn that sex—and love—can be joyful, liberating, and energizing.

Sensual Sex focuses on the present. As you begin to use all your senses during lovemaking, you will tap into the true ecstasy that can only come from feeling fully alive and being totally present in the moment.

Last, but certainly not least, Sensual Sex will provide you with a way to show your appreciation and gratitude for each other and to connect without the stress of expectations.

⑥ How This Book Is Organized ⑨

This book is divided into three parts. In part 1, "Sensual Joy," you'll be introduced to the concept of Sensual Sex and to the importance of sensuality and touch in relationships.

In part 2, "The Reawakening Your Senses Program," I offer the program that I designed to help couples and individuals become more aware of their senses. The Reawakening Your Senses Program is designed not only to reconnect you with your senses but also to teach you how to blend the sensual, the sexual, and the intimate. It will teach you how to relax so that you are more open to your senses, to sexual pleasure, and to your partner's expressions of love. It will reeducate you about how to give sensual pleasures, and, equally important, how to receive them. Finally, it will help you become more intimate, vulnerable, and trusting with your partner so that you can experience a deeper connection, one filled with ecstatic moments and life-transforming experiences.

In part 3, "The Four Seasons of Sensuous Passion," I offer suggestions and exercises for the four stages of an intimate, sexual relationship. Although all the techniques I provide in the book can be used by any couple at any time in their relationship, some are especially beneficial for particular age groups or at certain points in a relationship. Those who are starting out as a couple will learn positive habits that will ensure a long and healthy sexual life together. Those struggling to maintain a sexual relationship in the midst of raising children will learn how to be both a parent and a lover. Those going through midlife together will learn how to reassure their partners about their desirability and how to spice up their sex life after many years of marriage. Finally, those who are going through the stresses of aging will learn sensual, yet nonstressful, ways to comfort and show their love to each other.

⑥ Who the Book Is For ◎

Sensual Sex is for couples who would like to explore new ways of connecting both sexually and emotionally, couples who are not afraid to open themselves up to new experiences and new ways of loving. It will be especially beneficial to couples who would like to deepen their relationship and intensify their sensual and sexual feelings.

It is also for those individuals and couples who aspire to living a more conscious, fulfilling life, those who long for a deeper spiritual connection with each other.

Couples who are still getting to know each other will find that the exercises in this book will aid them in learning about each other's bodies, sexual preferences, and desires, while those who have been together a long time will find that the information and exercises offered here will help them to reconnect emotionally and physically and to regain the magic they felt together when they first fell in love.

Sensual Sex will also be of interest to couples who are currently experiencing relationship problems such as a lack of sexual desire, sexual incompatibility, or sexual dysfunction. Sex therapy or marital therapy can be quite expensive and is therefore beyond the reach of many people. *Sensual Sex* will provide many of the same things that a good sex therapist or marriage counselor can: accurate information, viable alternatives to your current way of relating, and exercises that will enhance your level of intimacy and arousal. Reading *Sensual Sex* will be like having a private sex therapist in your home.

Sensual Sex will offer specific help to couples who are trying to reconnect emotionally and sexually after their trust in each other has been betrayed (for example, if one or both partners have been unfaithful). Many of the exercises in the book will help these couples to reestablish trust and to rediscover their love for each other.

It will also benefit those who are starting over sexually, such as recovering alcoholics or those recovering from other addictions. People in Twelve-Step programs often find that once they experience sobriety, they begin to view sex in an entirely new way. *Sensual Sex* will offer a safe way to begin exploring both the joys and risks of intimacy, encouraging those in recovery to view sex from a far healthier perspective. It will encourage them to connect with their bodies, their senses, and their emotions instead of using sex to manipulate, to gain power, or to satisfy other needs. It will be especially helpful for people recovering from sex addiction.

Sensual Sex will also greatly benefit those who have been sexually abused as children or raped as adults. It will teach ways to make sex feel safe, help those who are shut down both sensually and sexually to open up once again to their senses, and offer couples a pleasurable way to connect emotionally and physically even when sexual intercourse is not an option. Reconnecting with one's senses and sensuality is especially important for people who have been sexually violated, because they need to gain a completely new perspective about sex to counter the negative effects of the abuse. For example, incest survivors are often robbed of the opportunity to experiment with their sensual and sexual feelings in ways that evolve naturally. Connecting with the joys of sensuality can help heal the shame associated with the body and sexuality that most survivors of sexual abuse experience.

Although I refer to a couple as "he and she," the information offered in *Sensual Sex* can also benefit homosexual couples who want to deepen their relationship or heal relationship wounds.

Last, but certainly not least, *Sensual Sex* will help couples who wish to forgo or postpone sexual intercourse. For example, those of you who wish to remain virgins until you marry will find that the sensuality exercises in the book offer you a viable alternative. The same holds true for those who find that they are unable or unwilling to engage in intercourse, such as those in the last stages of pregnancy, those with sexual dysfunctions, and those who are HIV-positive.

To summarize, *Sensual Sex* will be of benefit to:

❖ *couples who want to deepen their relationship and explore new areas of intimacy*

❖ *new couples who are just getting to know each other*

❖ *couples who want to reconnect emotionally and physically after years of perfunctory sex*

❖ *individuals and couples who have reached midlife and are experiencing the doubts, fears, and insecurities that come with facing aging bodies and hormonal changes*

❖ *older couples who wish to learn alternatives to strenuous sex*

❖ *couples who have become distant or estranged due to marital problems, extramarital affairs, or other situations that have eroded their trust*

❖ *people in recovery from substance abuse or other addictions, especially those in recovery from sex addiction*

❖ *couples in which one or both partners have histories of childhood sexual abuse*

❖ *couples in which one partner has recently experienced the trauma of rape*

❖ *people who wish to remain virgins until they get married*

❖ *those who are HIV-positive or have other medical problems that prevent them from engaging in intercourse.*

Although *Sensual Sex* is designed for couples, individuals can also benefit greatly from it. After all, sensuality begins with our own sensations and our own bodies. Throughout the book you will find exercises for you to do alone, either in preparation for a shared experience with your partner or as a way of enhancing your sexual experiences with your partner, even if he or she does not wish to cooperate.

⑥ Getting Your Partner Involved ⑥

Although some of you may be buying this book as a couple, most of you will be buying it in hopes of surprising your partner or enticing her or him into exploring more sensual ways of expressing your love for each other.

Thus, throughout the book you will be given suggestions for how to go about encouraging your partner's interest, including ways to gradually get a reluctant partner involved in the exercises. For example, if you invite your partner to do an exercise with you instead of expecting or demanding her to, she is far more likely to participate. Your invitation might be a handwritten note asking your partner to rendezvous in the bedroom at a particular hour. Or you could have some flowers delivered with a love note and an invitation to a special night out, during which you can broach the subject of adding more sensuality to your relationship. Some readers will undoubtedly give this book as a Valentine's Day or anniversary gift, a wonderful invitation in itself. Still another way to involve your partner would be to read a section or an exercise to him while you are lying in bed at night.

If you decide you'd like to read this book with your partner or to use the book as a starting point for conversations about your relationship, I suggest you sit down and talk to him about the reasons why you feel your relationship would benefit from *Sensual Sex*. If you decide to do so, start by reassuring your partner that you are still in love with him and by talking about all the good things about your relationship.

Sensual Sex will help couples to create and maintain a delightfully sensuous relationship, one that will stand the test of time and the stresses of modern life. Whether you are just beginning your relationship or have been together for many years, whether you are experiencing the bloom of youth or the comfort and acceptance of age, *Sensual Sex* will show you how to connect and reconnect with each other in a meaningful, yet joyful, way.

The more the soul knows,

the more she loves,

and loving much,

she tastes much.

— St. Catherine of Sienna

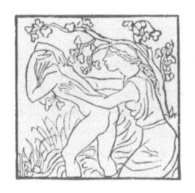

CHAPTER TWO

Our Hunger
for Sensuality
and Touch

W e all hunger for the healing tenderness of sensual touch, the soothing quality of sensual sounds and smells, and the titillation of sensual tastes. We yearn for the sweetness of intimacy. We long for a deeper connection with nature and with our souls. In fact, often our cravings for food, alcohol, drugs, and empty sex are really an attempt to satisfy our deep longing for these more meaningful and fulfilling desires and needs.

In this chapter I will address this hunger for sensuality and touch and begin setting the stage for helping you satisfy that hunger.

⑥ The Importance of Sensuality ⑥

Sensuality encompasses our enjoyment of and appreciation for how our bodies feel, and as such it is at the very heart of our sexuality. Our ability to receive and appreciate the pleasure our senses provide us with is intimately linked to our ability to be fully sexual. Without input from our senses, sex would be a very empty, perfunctory experience.

Think about the most exciting, arousing, satisfying sexual experience you have ever had. Try to recapture all the sensations you experienced—the feel of your skin against your partner's, the softness of your partner's lips, the intensity of your arousal and your partner's. Was visual stimulation a part of your experience? If so, remember the sights that added to your arousal and pleasure—the curve of your lover's body, the way his body glistened in the light, the expression of ecstasy on her face.

What other qualities made the experience so exciting? What other senses besides your sight were stimulated? Remember the love sounds you and your partner made together, the taste of her kisses, the smell of his skin.

Perhaps the setting itself added to your excitement or pleasure. If so, see in your mind's eye every detail of the scene. For example, if you were making love outside and this is what made the experience so special, recall every detail of your surroundings—the smell of the ocean or the pines, the feel of the sand or the earth against your skin, the sound of the ocean crashing or the trees whispering.

You are probably able to recapture far more of the experience when you engage your sense memory (your recollection of the senses that made up the experience). In fact, it is likely that it was your senses that made the experience so special in the first place, far more so than the quality of your orgasm or your partner's.

Sensuality is what distinguishes pure carnal sex from a loving, intimate bonding between two people. Touching, caressing, holding, and kissing are as important to lovemaking as the act of intercourse.

In addition to helping us become intimate and enhancing our sexual relationships, sensuality can serve as a viable alternative to intercourse. We all experience times when sexual intercourse is not possible (for example, during the latter months of pregnancy, because of illness, because of vaginal infections in women, because of erectile dysfunction in men, and because of the effects of aging). Therefore it is important that you be aware of and practice alternatives—sensual alternatives—to intercourse and other forms of lovemaking.

Sensuality also provides us with an important avenue for reconnecting or remaining connected with our bodies. The more connected you are with your own body, the more able you will be to connect with your partner's body, and the easier it will be to maintain a positive body image and to reach your orgasmic potential.

⑥ The Importance of Touch ⑥

All of life is a sensual experience, and yet most of us suffer from sensory deprivation. This is partly because we live in a highly sexual culture, yet one that is not very attuned to sensual pleasures. As a culture, we tend to focus on genital sex and to disregard the pleasures that other kinds of physical contact afford. Even lovers don't seem to touch as much as they want. Although this is usually not true in the beginning of a relationship, it is almost inevitable that once a relationship becomes sexual, the nonsexual touching that had previously been such an integral, pleasurable part of the relationship drops off sharply.

Unfortunately, the demands of our lives may deprive us of much of the physical contact that we once shared with each other and that we still need. We don't take time to touch each other. In some cases we are even afraid to touch one another. We're even running the risk of forgetting how to touch each other. Reaching out physically requires a vulnerability that many of us, in our attempts to be independent, self-contained, and successful, are in danger of losing. Many of us have learned to armor ourselves, to put up defenses in order to survive our stressful lives. Letting down these defenses, even when we are in the presence of our loved ones, can become increasingly difficult.

The importance of touch begins in childhood. Children who are cuddled and touched lovingly from the time they are born grow up to be well-adjusted adults able to establish and maintain healthy relationships. They have high self-esteem and, provided that other aspects of their upbringing were nurturing and that they didn't experience emotional, physical or sexual trauma, a healthy sense of their worth to others.

Conversely, the absence of touch and physical nurturing can create myriad problems. Infants and young children in orphanages, where they have little or no physical contact with other people, suffer from a condition once known as marasmus, what we now refer to as a "failure to thrive." These children are underweight, intellectually underdeveloped, and emotionally distant. Many die.

Those who were touch-deprived when they were young have a difficult time accepting loving touch as adults. Those not raised in a nurturing environment often have problems with their body image and their sense of worth.

As young children we instinctively reach out for pleasure in the form of love, comfort, and affection. If our needs are met lovingly and unconditionally, our capacity for pleasure survives and expands. But if our needs are met with criticism or rejection, pleasure becomes linked with pain and we may withdraw or develop defenses in order to reduce our anxiety.

Those of you whose parents believed in the importance of touch, who gave you adequate nurturing and caressing, have known the pleasures of physical touch both as a receiver and a giver. You know the importance of sensuality in your life—as a way to relax deeply and to express intimacy and love.

Those of you who were raised by parents who gave you very little physical nurturing, who may even have deprived you of physical touch, know firsthand how such deprivation can affect your self-esteem and ability to become intimate. Those who were not touched or who were taught that touch was dangerous (such as those whose parents rejected them when they reached out or those who were sexually abused) almost always grow up either afraid of touch and intimacy or so shut down that they cannot feel the pleasures of physical touch.

The good news is that we can reverse almost all the negative effects of touch deprivation. As a couple, you can help each other reclaim your natural capacity for pleasure through the use of sensual, loving touch. Together you can heal your childhood wounds, increase your potential for pleasure, and tear down the walls of defensiveness that have kept you feeling separate and alone.

And you can heal the wounds caused by deprivation experienced in adulthood as well. In most sexual relationships, touching and caressing play only a minimal role, a tremendous waste of our sensual potential and our potential for intimacy. Learning that our whole bodies can be erotic and increasing the amount of time you spend touching each other lovingly can deepen feelings of intimacy and greatly enrich and intensify your lovemaking. Many people find being caressed for an extended period of time even more intimate than lovemaking. Receiving intimate touch will help melt the armor that you have used to protect yourself and encourage you to share your feelings of anger, fear, and pain with each other. By daring to be vulnerable and free from rigid self-control, you will also free the flow of love between you.

Touch also has great potential as a healer of physical ailments. From the time of our birth to the day we die, we need to be touched to maintain emotional and physical health. From the nuzzles and caresses between mother and infant that form the foundation of the self, to the holding of hands between a son and his dying father that allows a final letting-go, touch is our most intimate and powerful form of communication. Just as it has been proven that children who receive adequate amounts of physical nurturing tend to develop better both emotionally and physically, research shows that couples who are affectionate with each other and who regularly connect physically (not necessarily sexually) tend to remain together far longer than those who have grown physically distant. It has also been shown that elderly people who regularly receive massages tend to become less depressed and to remain healthier than those who receive little or no touch, and that nursing-home patients who receive massages show fewer signs of senility.

Here are just a few of the many benefits of touch discovered by the latest research.

❖ *Cultures in which people express more physical affection toward infants and children tend to have lower rates of violence among adults.*

❖ *A simple touch can reduce the heart rate and lower blood pressure.*

❖ *Touch stimulates the brain to produce endorphins, the body's natural pain suppressers, which explains why when a mother hugs her child who has skinned his knee, she literally "makes it better."*

❖ *Studies have shown massage to have positive effects on conditions from colic to hyperactivity, from diabetes to migraines. It helps asthmatics to breathe easier, boosts immune function in HIV-positive patients, improves autistic children's ability to concentrate, lowers anxiety in depressed adolescents, and reduces apprehension in burn victims about to undergo debridement, the painful procedure in which contaminated skin is removed.*

❖ *Massage improves the body image of people suffering from eating disorders. As one recovering anorexic said, "I told myself that if this person thinks my body is okay enough to touch me, maybe my body is okay after all."*

❖ *Because massage stimulates the production of endorphins, touch can help prevent and treat addictive behaviors.*

Touch not only benefits the person receiving it but the one giving it as well. For example:

❖ *In a study in which volunteers over the age of 60 were given three weeks of massage and were then trained to massage toddlers at a preschool, giving massages proved even more beneficial than getting them. The elders exhibited less depression, lower stress hormone levels, and less loneliness. They made fewer visits to the doctor, drank less coffee, and called more friends on the phone.*

Many marital problems and most sexual problems can be healed through the magic of touch and sensuality. Certainly our deep sense of alienation and our feelings of emptiness can be alleviated when we learn to connect with each other on a deeper, more intimate level. Touch and sensuality offer an entrée to this more fulfilling level of relating as well as a way to strengthen and deepen already-existing levels of intimacy.

⑥ The Reawakening Your Senses Program ⑥

In the following chapters I will offer you my Reawakening Your Senses Program—exercises and information that will transform your way of thinking about sexuality, sensuality, and touch. Through this program you will not only learn how to be a better lover by replacing predictable, routine sex with Sensual Sex, but also how to satisfy your deep hunger for touch and sensuality. You will learn ways to connect with your partner on a more intimate level, thus ridding yourself of the alienation and emptiness that are all too common in our culture.

Among other things, by completing the Reawakening Your Senses Program you will learn:

❖ *how to awaken your senses and your natural sensuality*

❖ *how to deeply relax from the stresses of life and to melt into each other's arms*

❖ *how to touch your partner in a way that expresses your deepest love and appreciation and that also arouses sexual feelings that may have been dormant for a long time*

❖ *how to perceive your bodies as a playground for the senses, places to explore and experiment with, and to luxuriate in your sensations. You will begin viewing sex as an opportunity to be truly spontaneous. When this kind of spontaneity is present, your lovemaking will become an adventure—one that continues to bring new zest and thrill to your love life.*

❖ *how to connect with each other in a more deeply intimate way, a way that goes beyond words, expectations, and fears*

❖ *how to nurture your relationship, keeping it exciting, warm, and fulfilling*

❖ *how to be keenly aware of your own and your partner's body, so that every sensation becomes magnified and every bodily reaction is felt to the fullest.*

Once you have mastered these skills, you will be well on your way to becoming a more sensuous lover, and you will learn firsthand the multitude of rewards that Sensual Sex has to offer.

⊚ Before We Begin ⊚

The exercises that comprise the Reawakening Your Senses Program will ask you to set aside time for yourself and your relationship, time that may be hard to come by in your busy life. But if you don't set aside time now, you may find yourself becoming increasingly disconnected from your body and from your partner, which could lead to a growing lack of sexual desire, sexual problems, or emotional distancing from each other. Making a commitment to find the time, no matter how difficult, can be the best thing you ever do for your relationship.

You will undoubtedly find that the more time you spend reconnecting with your senses, the more time you will want to spend engaging in sensual and sexual pleasures. Even one hour a week spent in this pursuit could mean the difference between having an increasingly boring sex life and one that is full of pleasure, excitement, and joy. To get the most out of the exercises in this book, I encourage you to take some preliminary steps before embarking on the program. These include the following activities, explained in more detail below:

❖ *connecting with your inner sensor*

❖ *creating a sensory journal*

❖ *creating a sensory refuge*

❖ *developing a sensory mind-set*

Connecting with Your Inner Sensor—not Your Inner Censor

You will get far more out of this book and the Reawakening Your Senses Program if you begin with a mind-set of openness and curiosity, as opposed to one of skepticism and cynicism. You will never know whether a particular exercise will benefit you if you don't try it. Instead of discounting an idea or exercise because it sounds silly or because you feel self-conscious, approach each exercise with interest, enthusiasm, and a willingness to discover new things about yourself, your partner, and your relationship.

By connecting with your inner sensor, that is, your ability to sense, feel, and experience a particular situation or environment, instead of your inner censor, that part of you that stops you from sensing and feeling, that believes everything should be rational and logical, you will find that your sensual and sexual life will improve immensely.

Creating a Sensual Journal

As part of developing your inner sensor, begin a journal in which you detail your observations, reactions, and insights as you experience the various exercises in this book.

Begin your journal by writing about your personal hunger for more sensuality and touch in your life and how you feel your relationship and your life in general will benefit from the Awakening Your Senses Program. You may wish to share this with your partner as a way of encouraging her to participate in the program with you.

Then each time you complete an exercise, write about your reactions, including how each exercise made you feel, both physically and emotionally, and about any new awareness you may have about yourself, your partner, or your relationship.

Also write about any changes you feel the exercise will create in your relationship. Note what benefits and insights you experienced from the exercise, whether you felt closer to your partner or not, and which exercises you would choose to do again.

This last item will be especially beneficial later on after you've finished with the exercises and you and your partner begin to slip back into old habits. By going back to your journal and noting which exercises you liked the most, you may feel inspired to try them again. It will also spark your memory and hopefully your passions as you remember your reactions to an exercise the first time around.

Creating a Sensual Refuge

One of the most important preliminary steps to take before beginning the Awakening Your Senses Program is to create a sensual and erotic refuge—a private environment where you can go to explore and experiment with each other sensually and sexually, a place where you can find solace, strength, comfort, and deep union.

We all need a refuge from the noise, tension, and chaos of our daily lives. We all need a place to go where we can block out the intrusions and the pressures, where we can relax deeply and completely and become renewed and refreshed. One of the best ways to create greater intimacy and pleasure in your relationship is to create a sensual refuge where you can go individually and where you can meet as a couple.

Your sensual refuge should be a place where you can leave your worries behind, where you agree that there will be no talk of kids, work, or problems. It should be a place you make sacred by dedicating it to the express goal of nurturing your senses and renewing your relationship.

Creating such a refuge will serve as a physical reminder of your commitment to nurture each other, your relationship, and yourselves. Your sensual refuge can also offer a sense of hope and peacefulness. During times when you are too busy to spend much quality time together, just knowing your refuge is there and waiting for you will offer you hope and conjure up pleasant memories that can keep you going. In addition, your sensual refuge can serve as a neutral zone, a place where you can go in the midst of a conflict or unresolved argument.

Your sensual refuge should be a space where you are both comfortable and where you both have around you the things that will make you feel relaxed and sensual. To achieve this you will need to create your sensual refuge together. The following exercise will help you do this.

Exercise | Your Fantasy Refuge

Choose a time when you are both relaxed: sharing a glass of wine after the kids have gone to sleep, soaking in the hot tub or the bathtub together, lying in bed after making love or before going to sleep.

❖ *Take turns fantasizing out loud about where your ideal sensual refuge would be, what it would look like, and what you would do there together. Make sure you include all the sensory elements that would be important, all the smells, sounds, and sights that would make your refuge special. Again, don't let your inner censor get the better of you; instead, allow your inner sensor to take over. Let your imaginations run wild as you create just the right ambiance to both relax and titillate you. (Make sure you don't censor each other with derogatory comments or by making faces at each other's ideas.)*

❖ *Write down all the important elements of your fantasies. The ideal way to do this would be for you to take notes while your partner is talking, but if this isn't possible (because you are in the hot tub), do it as soon as possible.*

CREATING YOUR FANTASY REFUGE

Using your fantasies as a guide, find a space in your home where you can create a sensual refuge that contains at least some of the major elements of your fantasies. Decide which elements of your fantasies are the most important and try to incorporate them. For example, perhaps your partner said that his refuge would be in the woods—a cozy log cabin with a fire burning in the fireplace, an extremely quiet place except for the rustling of the pine trees outside. Even though you may live in a bustling urban area, you could create the illusion of a cabin by buying a plaid bedspread, putting up plaid curtains, installing a wood-burning stove, and adding some sprigs of pine or using pine scent.

Of course, it's possible that your fantasies are so different that you will find it difficult to combine them to create your refuge. If your fantasy is a beach hut on a tropical island, your husband's plaid bedspread and wood-burning stove could prove quite jarring. By working together you can agree on which elements are most important to each of you. For example, after some talking you may discover that what is really important to both of you is creating a feeling of nature in the room. You may decide to "marry" your tastes and create a nature refuge in which you both feel comfortable. Or you may agree to create more than one refuge, if space permits. The actual look of your refuge is less important than the mood it creates and the feelings it evokes when you are in it together.

If your partner does not wish to engage in the above exercise, you can still create your refuge using your own fantasy. Tell your partner that you would like to redecorate the bedroom and ask if he has any suggestions. If you have the kind of partner who says he doesn't care what you do, try incorporating some elements that you know would suit his personality and leaving out those that you know he wouldn't like.

The following suggestions will help you to create your fantasy refuge.

❖ *Redecorate the space you've chosen to reflect your desire to connect with your sensuality and sexuality. For example, choose soothing, sensual pictures or sexually stimulating ones. Fill the room with candles or place red or pink bulbs in your lamps. Change your lampshades, or put a dimmer on overhead lights.*

❖ *Get rid of distracting clutter that could prevent you from connecting with your sensuality.*

❖ *Put away reminders of former relationships or anything else that could elicit sad or angry feelings.*

❖ *Remove all reminders of work, including fax machines, computers, and files.*

❖ Experiment with various fragrances until you create an atmosphere that both of you can enjoy. Although some people like to set the mood by burning incense, the wrong incense can bring on allergic reactions, and the smokier varieties can create further irritation. In addition, since you will more than likely choose a scented oil for the caressing and massaging exercises, the different scents can conflict. (I will discuss choosing scented oils and essential oils in chapter 4.)

❖ Ensure your privacy by installing a lock on the door to your special place, removing answering machines, and unplugging or turning down the phone. If you are concerned about making noise, try improving the soundproofing by installing heavy drapes, putting down carpet, or lining the walls with bookshelves.

IMBUING YOUR SENSUAL REFUGE WITH LOVE AND RESPECT

To imbue your refuge with love and respect, first agree about how your refuge will be used and what behavior is or is not appropriate there. For example, you may wish to agree that your refuge be used as a neutral zone, meaning that there will be no arguing or mentioning subjects such as work or money. You may need to agree that you will not allow any interruptions once you are in your refuge together, such as answering the phone or the door.

You may wish to create a ceremony to designate your refuge as a special, sacred place. Your ceremony can include any number of rituals, including lighting candles, burning incense, mediating or praying together, or each of you saying a few words about your refuge and your relationship.

Some couples perform these rituals not only as part of a dedication ceremony but also each time they enter their sanctuary as a reminder of their purpose and dedication. Some hold hands and sing a song together, some read a poem out loud. These types of rituals can be especially effective if you use your refuge for other purposes throughout the day.

Developing a Sensual Mind-Set

Once you have prepared your special room, you will need to begin preparing your mind. Although many of the exercises in the book will help you to begin thinking and feeling in radically different ways, it's also important for you to begin to make the following changes now.

Retrain yourself to stay in the moment instead of slipping into fantasy. All too often when couples make love, one or both partners becomes lost in fantasy. This means, more times than not, that they are having sex with someone else. This not only deprives both partners of the deep satisfaction and feeling of intimacy that can come from emotionally connecting with each other but also cuts them off from the awareness of what is happening to their bodies.

For years now authors such as Nancy Friday have been telling us that it is okay to fantasize while we're making love. We've been given permission to imagine we are having sex with someone else, anyone else, as long as it turns us on. After all, we are told, it doesn't hurt our partners. We are told that since the brain is the most erogenous organ in the body, all sex begins there anyway, and that any fantasy, no matter how wild, can do us no harm.

But this is not entirely true. Fantasy takes us away from the moment and away from our partner. How can we hope to feel intimate with our partner when we aren't even there? Put simply, if you are making love to a fantasy person you aren't making love to your partner. You aren't emotionally or spiritually available.

The brain is the most erotic part of the body only if we are cut off from the rest of our body, our emotions, and our sensuality. If, however, we are connected to these important parts of ourselves, it is our skin that is our most erotic organ. After all, our skin is the point of contact with our partner, the part of our body that provides us with the greatest feelings of connectedness, nurturing, and sensual and sexual pleasure. If we are lost in fantasy we also cut off from much of the pleasure our skin can provide.

Focus on staying in your body instead of in your head. Many of us tend to be so tense and preoccupied with our daily struggles that we have a difficult time turning off our minds when we make love. Our worries creep in at the most inopportune moments. As a way of helping you to stay in the moment and out of your head, I encourage you to retrain yourself to focus all your attention on the point of contact between your body and that of your partner's at any given time. Therefore, if you are kissing your partner, all your focus will be on how your lips feel against your partner's, the feel of her tongue as it plays with yours, and how the kiss makes your body feel. You aren't worrying about whether you have bad breath. Nor are you allowing your mind to jump forward to what you want your partner to do next, or to what you need to do the next day.

If your partner is caressing your back, all your attention is focused on how his touch feels on your body, all the exquisite sensations you are experiencing. You aren't thinking about how your partner feels, whether he is getting tired, or whether the kids will be home soon.

If you are caressing your partner's thighs, you are focusing all your attention on the point of contact between your hand and your partner's body. You aren't jumping forward to what you are going to do next or worrying about whether your touch is turning your partner on sufficiently.

Focus on sensuality instead of performance. Today, more than ever, the pressure is on for both men and women to be physically perfect and sexually superior. People in relationships worry about whether they are physically appealing, whether they are sexually exciting, and whether they can satisfy each other. Men worry about their erections and how long they will last, while women worry about whether they can have an orgasm, and even if they can have multiple orgasms.

If you are worried about whether you are pleasing your partner, you are not completely present and therefore cannot fully experience your bodily sensations. If all your energy is focused on watching your partner's reactions, you will not be able to focus sufficiently on your own and you will not be aware of your senses.

By the same token, if you are anxious
about whether you will have an orgasm
or whether you will be able to with-
hold it, you will miss the pleasurable
sensations your body is experiencing. Many sexual problems are actually caused by the anxiety created by
the pressure to perform. This type of
anxiety creates both tensions in the
body and shallow breathing, which in
turn can interfere with your natural sexual
arousal response.

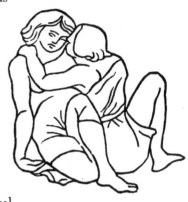

Sensual Sex is about being as aware as possible of every nuance of feeling your body is experiencing, of the sights, sounds, smells, and tastes
involved in the act of lovemaking. When you are able to achieve this intense
focus you will be able to block out distractions, extraneous thoughts, or
preoccupations. You will be so caught up in pleasure that worrying about
performance will seem superfluous.

When both partners in a relationship can achieve this kind of focus the
results are incredible. A great freedom comes from knowing that your partner is not focused on your pleasure or your orgasm. It takes the burden off
you to perform or to please your partner. When you know that your partner is just as caught up in experiencing the pleasure of your bodies coming
together, just as caught up with his or her senses, you can relax and stop
worrying about pleasing.

Perhaps this advice to focus on your own feelings and sensations instead
of your partner's sounds as if I am suggesting that you become selfish and
less caring. This couldn't be farther from the truth. Worrying about
whether you are pleasing your partner or whether your partner is close to
orgasm doesn't help her experience more pleasure. In fact, research con-
sistently shows that those who are aware of their partner's concern are usually more inhibited and less able to relax than those who do not have this
added pressure. And focusing all your attention on your partner's orgasm

certainly doesn't add to your own pleasure. More than likely you will begin to tire or get bored, and you may even become irritated with your partner if he doesn't reach an orgasm in a reasonable amount of time.

Think about the last time you focused all your attention on your partner's orgasm. Even though you may love your partner and want to please her, didn't it begin to feel more like a task than a pleasure at some point? And once your partner reached orgasm, did you really feel that close to each other? Your partner may have felt grateful to you for your persistence, and you may have felt relieved and happy for your partner. But did you feel deeply connected? Focusing on sensuality instead of performance will help you to deepen your relationship. Paradoxically, the more you focus on your own pleasure and senses, the more you will be able to surrender to deeper feelings of love for your partner. This is true for several reasons.

First, the more pleasure you allow yourself to feel (without the restrictions of guilt or performance anxiety), the better you will feel about yourself. The better you feel about yourself, the more loving you are likely to feel toward your partner.

Second, by focusing on your own pleasure you will learn more about what you enjoy, and this will make it easier to communicate these desires to your partner.

Third, while it is normal to want to please your partner and to add to his enjoyment, focusing on your own sensations and your own enjoyment will actually make you more sensitive to your partner's needs and feelings. This is because the more in touch you are with your own body, the more attuned you will become to your partner's. Eventually, you will become so attuned to your partner's body that you will almost be able to feel her reactions as well. Ultimately, your partner's pleasure will become yours.

Finally, by removing performance pressure from your relationship you free yourself and your partner to surrender to feelings of vulnerability and love. This is because the more pleasure we experience, the more vulnerable we become. Opening up to each other this way, although initially frightening, can create a tremendously strong bond between you, a bond that few other experiences can create.

Slow down. Learning to slow down, to stop rushing through lovemaking and instead to luxuriate in every sensation may be difficult at first. We are used to rushing to get into bed together, rushing to have an orgasm or to help our partner reach one, and then lying together feeling empty and unsatisfied and wondering why.

Slowing down is one of the most important actions you can take to create a more satisfying sexual relationship, because it will encourage you to connect with yourself and your partner in a more meaningful way. Rushing toward orgasm can actually be a way of avoiding intimacy. Taking the time to experience your sensations and to experience each other, however, encourages and nurtures intimacy.

To remind yourself to *slow down,* repeat the words slow down like a mantra during each of the touching exercises in the book. Even when you think you are going slow enough you probably are not, at least in the beginning, so slow down even more.

Be open to new experiences. It is often difficult to be open to new experiences. We become afraid, we feel self-conscious. It takes courage and determination to confront and overcome these feelings, yet think of the alternatives. You could remain as you are, safely nestled in the security of routine sex, or you could venture out a little bit to discover what lies beyond. Your current sex life, while providing the comforts of a well-worn shoe, offers no surprises and probably doesn't encourage you to explore and discover a deeper relationship. The beauty of being open to Sensual Sex is that you don't have to worry about losing anything. You will only add to your relationship, not take anything away. Learning to engage in Sensual Sex is like shopping for new shoes when you already have plenty of comfortable ones in the closet.

Learning these new attitudes and behaviors may seem difficult or awkward at first, but you will find that, as with any new behavior, the more you practice them, the more natural they will begin to feel.

My goal is to have these new attitudes and behaviors become an integral part of your life. Throughout this book I offer you a series of exercises designed specifically to help you with this process. The Reawakening Your Senses Program presented in part 2 will begin the process by offering information and exercises to awaken your senses, connect with your partner through sensuous touch, immerse yourself in the sensuality of water and massage oils, and discover the surprising joy of sacred sex.

It is my firm belief that increasing the amount of sensuality and touch in your relationship can and will do more for it than any other single factor. When you give yourself and your partner the gift of sensuality, you will not only change your relationship for the better but you will also improve the rest of your lives. Sensuous people are connected to their feelings, their environment, and their bodies more intensely than other people are. Sensuous people are more in tune with others' feelings, and they have a far greater chance of connecting with their partners in an authentic, intimate, rewarding way. Sensuous couples enjoy a far more loving, intimate, and exciting sex life than other couples, and they stay together longer and ultimately experience more pleasure and more happiness.

Part II

❖   ❖   ❖

The Reawakening Your Senses Program

The moment one gives close attention

to anything, even a blade of grass,

it becomes a mysterious, awesome,

indescribably magnificent world in itself.

– HENRY MILLER

Here are fruits, flowers, leaves

and branches,

And here is my heart which beats

only for you.

– "CHANSON D'AUTOMNE," PAUL VERLAINE

CHAPTER THREE

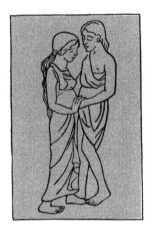

Reconnecting with Your Five Senses

An exciting and fulfilling sexual experience involves far more than the intensity of the orgasm or even the sexual act itself. It involves all our senses. The feel of your lover's skin as you slowly caress and explore it. The intense intimacy of your lover's body pressed up against yours. The heat generated by your movements and your emotions. The pungent sex smells. The occasional glimpse in a mirror or out of the corner of your eye of your lover's body, or of your bodies dancing together to the rhythm of your love. The intimate taste of your kisses, the salty flavor of your lover's excited skin. The sounds of your lovemaking—the moans and sighs that bespeak your lover's pleasure, the cries of surrender.

Unfortunately, most of us don't pay enough attention to the myriad messages our senses send us. We therefore deprive ourselves of the kinds of sensual and sexual experiences we all deserve and miss out on so much of what life has to offer. This chapter provides you with exercises specially designed for each of your five senses, exercises that will help you to develop your sensory awareness. By increasing your responsiveness and sensitivity you can open up a whole new sensual way of being and begin to feel more in touch with the world around you. By expanding your sensual awareness you can become more attuned to your own body and your partner's and together develop an increasingly erotic relationship.

⑥ Developing Your Senses ⑥

Our senses are our point of contact with the world. They bring us information about what is around us and provide us with a way to experience the world with immeasurable pleasure.

Unfortunately, much of our sensing ability lies dormant, unused and unappreciated. You only need to remember the times when your senses were heightened by an unusual circumstance to fully appreciate what I am saying. Think back to when you first fell in love. You were no doubt keenly aware of your environment. Colors were more intense, birds seemed to sing louder, flowers seemed to be more fragrant. You probably felt more alive than at any other time in your life.

Something similar happens when we are on vacation. Away from the tasks that take us from our senses we tend to pay more attention to the sights, sounds, smells, and textures around us. At such times we feel relaxed and more fully in the here and now. Our senses are also heightened when we are in the midst of change. Moving to a new house or starting a new job can get us to take note of our environment far more than during ordinary times. Suddenly we notice how beautiful the trees that line our street are.

In our day-to-day lives, however, our senses are often dulled. We seldom take the time to experience our environments in a fully observant way. Although the senses themselves never cease to pick up and relay information, we perceive only what we pay attention to. If our minds are preoccupied, we miss most of the messages our senses are sending us. We become more like machines than people, rushing back and forth between work and home, our minds consumed with tasks and problems, our bodies and sensory impressions forgotten.

Our senses are also greatly affected by our feelings. We often escape from the painfulness of reality by blunting our senses. Sometimes we do this unconsciously, while at other times we deliberately block things out, such as not looking at the homeless people on the street or not responding to angry or painful words spoken by others.

Moreover, our sensory systems are tuned to recognize and screen out normal, familiar stimuli and to bring to our notice only what seems unusual or threatening to our survival, such as footsteps on the stairs, a rotten smell, an unfamiliar taste. This sensory screening is essential, for without it we would be drowned in a flood of sensation and would find it difficult to cope with daily tasks. Those of us who live in a crowded city, for example, would become totally overwhelmed by sounds, smells, and sights.

As a result of our sensory-screening ability, we also miss many of life's gifts—seeing what is around us, tasting all the subtle flavors in our food, noticing all the sounds that make up the symphony of life.

When operating at their full capacity, our senses are extraordinarily finely tuned, able to pick up even the most subtle distinctions. By just touching her child's forehead, a mother can tell whether his body temperature has deviated by more than a degree or two from normal. People who study music can distinguish between a half and a quarter tone in music, while some rose experts can distinguish a rose just by its smell.

✆ Awakening to Your Natural Sensuality ✆

Becoming more sensual is really more about not continuing to rob yourself of your natural sensuality than it is about learning anything new. As children we were all naturally sensual. In fact, children can teach adults a lot about noticing their environment—about paying attention to colors, sounds, and the other textures of life. Notice how small children use all their senses to explore their environment. They "absorb" their environment by smelling, tasting, touching, seeing, and listening. Watch small children explore a new object. First they look at it, taking in every nuance of color. Then they feel the texture and shape of it. Before long they are shaking it near their ears, smelling it, or licking it. They have fully immersed themselves in exploring it using all their senses. Now think about the last time you came anywhere close to exploring your environment in this way.

Although we are all born with the ability to use and appreciate our senses, all too often our attention to the sensuous was diverted when we were young children. Continually told that we shouldn't put things in our mouth or that we shouldn't touch them, we soon stopped exploring the world as fully as we once did.

You can retrain yourself to open up once again to your surroundings, to regain this natural appreciation of your senses. Begin by taking advantage of potentially sensuous activities like eating, bathing, and dressing instead of treating them as routine chores. For example, if you rush in and out of the shower to save time, you are robbing yourself of the chance to relax in the warm water and feel its sensual play on your skin. You could make meal-times a time for sensual enjoyment, allowing yourself plenty of time to explore. Learn to enjoy the different textures of food: crunchy, smooth, grainy. (Notice how toddlers who are newly introduced to food spend more time playing with it than eating it.)

Here are some other suggestions.

❖ *If you have a dog or cat, pay attention to how soft its fur is, how the fur has different textures in various parts of your pet's body.*

❖ *Pull the petals off a rose. Feel their softness against your skin, on your lips.*

❖ *Listen to a variety of new types of music. We become so acclimated to familiar music that we don't notice the nuances. See how many different instruments you can hear. Notice how the music makes you feel.*

The following two exercises will help you to continue exploring your senses. Don't allow your inner censor to discourage you from this exploration by convincing you that it is silly or a waste of time. There's nothing silly about your sensuality, about your ability to experience life and love to the fullest.

You will notice that in addition to helping you to develop your sensory awareness, many of these exercises will also encourage you to pay attention to how experiencing your senses makes you feel emotionally. This is because being open to your senses is a crucial part of your ability to be open to intimacy and love. Just as we close off our senses as a self-protective measure to block out unwanted stimuli, we also close them off to block out uncomfortable emotions and to protect ourselves from becoming too intimate.

Exercise | **The Nature Walk**

There was a time, not so long ago, when our very survival depended upon our being keenly attuned to nature. Remaining alive meant daily wandering, searching, and exploring of the surrounding world. For example, as Australian Aborigines walked through the countryside, they repeatedly stopped and tasted the fruit of unfamiliar plants, smelled their leaves, dug out and examined roots, broke and examined stems, and tasted and smelled the sap, often rubbing it on their bodies. They observed intensely any bird, animal, or insect in their vicinity.

They carried out this sensory exploration almost automatically, and as they walked they shared information with one another about the medicinal and ritual value of plants and food.

Although our survival no longer depends on how observant we are in nature, our sensuality can be greatly enhanced by following the example of our ancestors and by keenly observing our environment, to appreciate texture, flavor, fragrance, hue, timbre, and more.

Preparation: For this exercise, imagine that you are living in an undeveloped society in which your very life depends on your ability to observe your surroundings. If at all possible, choose a rugged, isolated environment, or at least someplace where you won't feel self-conscious about exploring your senses and where you won't be disturbed by passersby. You can do this exercise alone or with your partner. Pay attention to how this experience makes you feel, both sensually and emotionally.

1. As you walk around, closely observe every tree and bush you come upon. Feel the bark of the trees with your hands, pick a leaf and feel its texture and then sniff it to see if it has a smell. Pick a flower or bud, feel its smoothness against your fingertips, crush it between your fingers to smell its fragrance.

2. If you come across an animal, pay close attention to its features, the colors of its hide or fur, the way it moves, the sounds it makes. Pay attention to whether it has a noticeable smell. Do the same with any insects or birds you see.

3. Feel the texture of the ground underneath you and notice when the terrain changes. Dig a hole in the dirt or sand. Notice if there are any insects hidden there. Feel the texture of the dirt or sand, let it run through your fingers, squeeze it together in your fist and see if it holds together.

E x e r c i s e | **The Sensory Basket**

Collect a variety of objects that you find pleasurable to touch, smell, taste, listen to, or look at, such as satin cloth, polished rocks, feathers, flower petals, fruit, bells, and jewelry. Put your objects in a basket, bowl, or special box. Spend a few minutes focusing on each object. Hold each object, feel its texture, smell it, taste it, or listen to it. Decide which are your favorites. Now share your basket with your partner.

Keep your basket by your bedside or in your bathroom as a reminder to stay aware as you go about your daily life. Or you could keep a small sensory basket on your desk at work as a reminder to stop and play and feed your senses periodically throughout your day.

In the following pages you will be introduced to more ways to reconnect with each of your five senses. We will focus on one sense at a time, encouraging you to become more aware of your environment by focusing on this particular sense only. Then you will be encouraged to use all your senses together to have a complete experience.

⊚ Sight ⊚

Sight is often our most dominant sense, perhaps because the eyes, like the ears, are extensions of the brain. This is true in spite of the fact that the sense of touch may exceed the sense of sight in the numbers of signals sent to the brain.

We rely on sight more than on any other sense to teach us about our environment. Try paying attention to only what your eyes are doing for a minute or two. You will notice that they ceaselessly jump about from one point to another, never remaining still. What we observe through our eyes is like a series of snapshots. It is from this collection of impressions that we build an overall impression of our environment.

Unlike animals who "sniff out" danger, our sense of sight helps us determine whether a situation or a person is "safe" or not. If an environment is displeasing to the eye, we tend to reject it right away without waiting to find out if it pleases our other senses. The same is true of the people we meet. Although our sight was initially developed to protect us from danger, it also helps us determine who we will connect with and who we won't. Whether we like it or not, if people are unattractive to us, especially if they have physical features that are displeasing to us for whatever reason, we are less open to them and have a more difficult time connecting emotionally with them. The same holds true for whether people will be sexually attractive to us or not.

Even though we rely so strongly on sight, we see only a small portion of what is around us. There are so many nuances, so many details that we miss. The world is full of colors, shapes, and textures that go unnoticed as we go about our busy lives. Therefore, by reawakening your sense of sight you will add depth, interest, and excitement to your life and you will make your love life far more fulfilling.

Exercise | **Consciously Seeing**

In the exercises that follow, you will practice focusing your attention primarily on what you see, making your sense of sight more acute while muffling your other senses.

1. Begin to notice your immediate environment—colors, shapes, and textures—as if you were seeing it for the first time. Take a close look at the inside of your house. Notice the various colors, shapes, and textures that create your environment. Now go for a walk and open your eyes to what is around you. Rediscover the beauty in the commonplace. If you live in the city, notice the architecture, the different colors and shapes of the billboards, the people of all shapes and sizes. If you live in the suburbs or the country, pay attention to the color of the sky, the different varieties of trees and flowers, the various textures of the ground you are walking on.

When you come upon something that catches your eye because it is beautiful, don't just rush by. Linger for a moment and take in its beauty. Notice that sometimes something can be so beautiful that we are unable to look at it for very long. Why do you think this is? Intense beauty stirs up deep feelings inside us—it touches our soul. Those of us who are used to being cut off from these deep feelings may find this experience uncomfortable. It can be painful to open ourselves to beauty just as it can be painful to open ourselves to love. If you notice that you cannot keep your eyes on an object of beauty or a beautiful scene in nature for very long, allow yourself to look away, but then take a deep breath and try looking at it again. Continue breathing and see if you can continue taking in the beauty a little longer this time.

2. Now observe your partner as if you were seeing her for the first time. Notice every detail of your partner's face and body—her skin, hair, each feature on her face, each limb of her body.

    How do you feel when you do this? Is there a part of your partner's body that makes you feel uncomfortable when you look at it? Why do you think this is? Are there parts of your partner's body that are so beautiful that it is painful to take them in completely?

    If there is a part of your partner's body that you find unattractive, notice your negative reaction or judgment and then move your eyes to a part of his body you find very attractive.

    Remember when you first met your partner and how you reacted to his appearance at the time. Has your reaction changed? Do you still find your partner as attractive as you once did? If not, this could be a symptom of the distance that has developed between you, either because of neglect or pent-up feelings.

3. Finally, instead of closing your eyes the next time you make love, open them so that you can take in your partner. Really look at your partner's face and body as you make love. Watch yourself in the act of making love. Notice how difficult it can be to do this. Although it may be uncomfortable to be so vulnerable, you will find that by

keeping your eyes open you will stay more focused on the present and will eventually be able to reach greater levels of physical pleasure and deeper levels of intimacy with your partner.

Exercise | **Enhancing Your Sexuality Through Your Sense of Sight**

Your sense of sight can greatly add to your sexual pleasure. We used to believe that men were more highly sensitive to visual stimulation than women, but recent research shows that women are keenly sensitive to visual stimulation too, and that it enhances their arousal. The following suggestions will help you discover just how sensitive you are and will help you find ways to add excitement to your love life.

❖ *Experiment with lighting to discover whether you prefer to make love in the dark or whether you become more aroused by looking at your partner's naked body. The sight of aroused genitals, your bodies being physically joined together, or your lover approaching and reaching orgasm can be especially exciting. Try a variety of lighting such as candles, different colored light bulbs, or scarves placed over lamp shades to create various moods. If it turns out that one of you likes the lights on while the other prefers them off, a compromise can be reached with dim lighting.*

❖ *Some people, women as well as men, find watching themselves as they make love highly erotic, so hanging mirrors in your room may enhance your lovemaking.*

❖ *Looking deep into each other's eyes as you make love is a wonderful way of maximizing sensual pleasure and emotional intimacy.*

❖ *Experiment with sexy lingerie or sexy pajamas or underwear.*

⑥ Hearing ⑥

Our sense of hearing provides us with the greatest capacity to take in what is happening around us. Without it we would be radically cut off from our environments. Moreover, sound can have a tremendous effect on our mood. Sounds such as children screaming, phones ringing, or horns honking can make us tense, nervous, and irritated, while sounds such as soft music, waves gently lapping at the shore, or the wind rustling through the trees can be soothing. Sounds can also elicit memories from the past— the sound of a train whistle in the distance can make you feel nostalgic for your childhood, the sound of a siren can remind you of a car accident you were in.

Music can be particularly powerful in affecting our mood and stirring up memories. It can calm us when we are stressed, lift our spirits when we are down, and help us to express emotions that are difficult to communicate. Music has been found to lower blood pressure and the level of stress hormones in our blood. It has been used in medical and psychiatric settings to do everything from helping cancer patients to endure chemotherapy to lifting depression in the elderly. It can also stir the libido and help "get you in the mood."

According to research women tend to respond to sound more intensely than men. It is uncertain whether they actually hear better or if they are just more distracted by sound. The slightest sound can grab a woman's attention during lovemaking, whereas men can become so involved that they don't seem to hear even loud sounds.

Our hearing can be remarkably selective. It sorts out what we want to hear from what we would rather not, what we need to hear from what we don't. Unfortunately, since most of us are bombarded with unwanted sounds all day long, we begin to lose some of the acuteness of our hearing. We can regain this acuteness by paying attention to the sounds around us.

Exercise | **Consciously Hearing**

The following exercises will help awaken your sense of hearing and make you more attuned to your surroundings.

1. Begin by noticing all the obvious sounds around you—the sounds of cars going by, of dogs barking, of children playing. Pay attention to how these sounds make you feel. Notice how effective our sensory system is in screening out annoying and distracting sounds. Now listen for the less obvious sounds—the ticking of the clock, the chirping of the birds outside. Notice how these sounds make you feel and what you have been missing by not taking the time to listen to them.

2. Go with your partner to a location where you can experience nature together. Notice the sounds of nature all around you—the water gently lapping on the shore, the seagulls calling, the trees rustling in the wind. Pay attention to the sounds you and your lover make—the crunch of dried leaves under your feet, your breathing as you walk, your lover's voice and laughter.

3. Finally, notice the sounds your lover makes when you are making love. Taking in your lover's sounds in this way can create a feeling of intense intimacy and can become quite arousing. Now notice the sounds you make together. This may be a little more difficult because you may feel self-conscious, but keep trying. Once you get past your self-consciousness you may find that these sounds are also very arousing. Do the sounds you make fully express how you are feeling? By listening to the sounds you both make while making love, and by expressing yourself through sounds, you may find yourself experiencing a deepened sexual connection with your partner.

E x e r c i s e | **Enhancing Your Sexuality**
Through Your Sense of Hearing

Try the following suggestions to see if they intensify the sexual pleasure you experience with your partner.

❖ *Make a point of deliberately expressing your feelings for your lover through sounds only instead of words.*

❖ *If your lover touches you in an especially pleasurable way, allow yourself to moan in response.*

❖ *When you touch your lover erotically, signal your enjoyment by purring or by making a throaty sound.*

❖ *Don't underestimate the power of music to stir up passionate feelings or to remind you of when you were first together. The right music can help even when you're tired or uninterested.*

Bring a tape recorder or CD player into the bedroom and explore music's potential to relax, soothe, and excite you. Experiment with various types of music or nature sounds to bring out the savage beast in you both. Take turns choosing music that will set the kind of mood you would like to experience together sexually. Take some risks. In addition to choosing classics like Ravel's *Bolero,* experiment with albums by the group Enigma or with primitive music and music from other cultures—African drum music, East Indian sitar music, and calypso music—music that is playful, passionate, or deeply emotional. If you are looking for intensity, try Wagner. If you want to get swept away, try environmental recordings such as *Ultimate Thunderstorm.* For New Age erotic music, try the sensual *Moments in Love* from *The Best of the Art of Noise.*

Take a trip to a music store together and find music that best expresses your love for each other. Here are some suggestions.

Try *Scheherazade* by Rimsky-Korsakoff, Mozart's 21st Piano Concerto, *Rapture* by Anita Baker, *Love Deluxe* by Sade, anything by Chet Baker. As far as oldies are concerned, how about, *The First Time*

Ever I Saw Your Face by Roberta Flack, *Sexual Healing,* by Marvin Gaye, *Can't Help Falling in Love with You,* by Elvis, anything by the Platters, and almost anything by Johnny Mathis.

⑥ Smell ⑥

Smell is the most evocative of our senses, capable of changing our mood and bringing back memories. Yet it is also the most ignored, its powerful messages often passing us by unnoticed.

We take in smells subliminally all the time. These subliminal odors cause us to feel uncomfortable in some surroundings and comfortable in others; they cause us to like or dislike a person; they even have a great effect on who we fall in love with.

Each person has his or her own "personal scent," just as we have unique fingerprints, with no two people's being exactly alike. Newborn babies are able to identify their mothers by smell, as can couples (although often unconsciously).

Kissing is one of the best ways for us to intimately "smell" each other. In fact, the word *kiss* means "to smell" in several languages. The face has many sweat glands, which play a key role in producing a person's characteristic smell. Other areas of the body that have a large number of sweat glands are considered erogenous zones. It is primarily these areas, and the odors produced there, that make up the smell characteristic to each person.

Women generally have a keener sense of smell than men, especially when they are ovulating. It isn't any surprise, then, that women tend to have stronger reactions to certain body odors, such as perspiration and bad breath. Though many women are offended by the smell of a man's sweaty body, some are actually aroused by it. Scents that are similar to men's sexual musk can also be highly arousing to women. Men tend to react more negatively to artificial scents, especially those that are sprayed freely around the house, such as room deodorizers.

Exercise | **Consciously Smelling**

The following exercises will help to reawaken your sense of smell.

1. Gather together some strong-smelling objects—flowers, fresh or dried herbs, peeled and cut fruit, soap, and so on. Close your eyes, and picking up one object at a time, slowly absorb its fragrance. Notice how each scent makes you feel.

2. Try making a meal on the basis of smell. Include a succession of dishes, ranging from pungent to bland, and inhale the smell of each dish before eating it.

3. Pay attention to how your partner smells throughout the day. Notice the way his skin smells right after a morning shower versus how he smells at the end of the day. Pay attention to the fragrances she uses and how the scents of different body-care products affect her overall smell. Notice how different foods, alcohol, cigarette or cigar smoke also affect how she smells.

   Notice how each scent creates an internal, emotional, and sometimes even a physical reaction in you. For example, when your partner comes out of the shower smelling sweet and clean, it may cause your heart to melt and make you feel like embracing him; whereas when he comes home after a busy day at work with the smell of car exhaust permeating his skin from his long drive on the freeway, you may feel sorry for him but not as inclined to hug him. After he's been out with the boys drinking and smoking cigars you may not only feel repulsed by his smell but angry as well.

   Notice, too, how certain bodily smells can elicit strong memories. For example, does your heart pound with excitement every time your wife wears a certain fragrance because it reminds you of when you were first together? Does your husband's sweat arouse you or repulse you? Does the smell of alcohol on your lover's breathe turn you on, or conversely, turn you off because it brings

up memories of an alcoholic family member? Now notice your partner's body smells during sex and whether these smells elicit positive
or negative feelings in you. Pay attention to these feelings and see if
you can connect them to any memories.

Exercise | Enhancing Your Sexuality
Through Your Sense of Smell

According to Valerie Gennari Cooksley in her book *Aromatherapy:
A Lifetime Guide to Healing With Essential Oils,*

*the importance of the olfactory system and its role in sexuality is plain to see.
It is known that anosmia or hyposmia (an absent or decreased ability to smell)
has been associated with a decreased interest in sex.... Our sense of smell is
very important in our lives, especially in the sexual arena. In fact, as many as
25% of the people who experience smell disorders also lose interest in sex.*[1]

To enhance your lovemaking try the following exercises:

1. Since the association between smell and emotions is extremely powerful, we are becoming more and more aware of how therapeutic it
   is to smell good smells—freshly baked breads, roasting coffee beans,
   forest pine. Sit down together and share with each other which
   smells turn you on. Once again, don't let your inner censor prevent
   you from being open with each other. Recent research has actually
   uncovered the fact that men tend to become sexually aroused by the
   scent of baked goods! Many people find the scent of perspiration,
   vaginal lubrication, or semen highly erotic, while others are repulsed
   by these smells.

2. The purpose of this exercise is to discover which artificial scents are
   sexually arousing to each of you. Begin by gathering all the fragrances
   you currently use, including perfumes, aftershaves, soaps, lotions,
   scented candles, incense, and room deodorizers. Individually take a
   whiff of each scent and eliminate any that particularly offend you.
   Once you have both done this, each of you choose one scent that is

your favorite, one that you would like to include as an entré into your lovemaking or as part of your lovemaking.[2]

3. We'll discuss the benefits of essential oils, as well as how to use them, in the next chapter, but for now, go to a store that carries massage and essential oils and choose a scent that you both enjoy, one that feels particularly "sexy" to each of you. Buy either a bottle of scented massage oil that has this scent or an essential oil from which you can create your own massage oil. At home, add some of the essential oil to a bottle of unscented massage oil until you reach the desired concentration. Now give each other a massage using your special oil.

⑥ Taste ⑥

Our sense of taste may not have the impact on our sexual lives that some of our other senses do, but it definitely affects our sexuality. This is partly because our senses of taste and smell are inextricably linked. When we smell something appetizing, our mouth automatically begins to water, and when we smell something rotten we get a bad taste in our mouth. If you like how your partner smells, it can whet your appetite for kissing, fondling, and tasting more of her.

Another reason why our sense of taste affects our sex life is that anything we do with our mouth has the double effect of stimulating both our sense of taste and our sense of touch. When you taste something, your mouth is also being stimulated, which in turn can elicit sexual feelings. More than likely, you, like most people, have at some point become aroused by eating sensuous food such as sushi or figs or other fruit.

Sucking and licking are oral pleasures that everyone experiences. Whether you are sucking and licking on a popsicle, a lollipop, a finger, or your lover's genitals, you are likely to become aroused sexually.

Exercise | **Tasting with Awareness**

Awakening to the power of taste can greatly enhance your sex life, as well as the rest of your life. Begin to do this by reducing input from the other senses, especially your sight, focusing your attention on the sense of taste only. The following exercises will help.

1. Prepare a meal for yourself, choosing foods that appeal to all areas of the palate—sweet, salty, sour, bitter, and savory. For example, choose succulent fruits that are sweet, sour, and bitter; choose crackers that are salty and savory. Begin to eat the food slowly, relishing the flavor of every mouthful. Enjoy the process of biting, chewing, and swallowing. Notice how your teeth and tongue interact with the food. Pause occasionally as you eat, and notice if the taste changes as the food is broken down. Swallow slowly. You may be surprised at how full you feel before you complete your meal. Most of us eat only to "fill our bellies," not really to experience the richness and variety of taste sensations our food can provide. In fact, many believe that if we consciously tasted and smelt what we eat, we wouldn't eat as much.

2. Notice the way your partner's skin tastes: its saltiness, the way various parts of her body taste different. Notice how his kisses taste to you at various times and the different feelings this can arouse.

Exercise | **Enhancing Your Sexuality**
Through Your Sense of Taste

❖ *Experiment with sucking, licking, and nibbling various parts of your lover's body. Feel free to experiment and explore new territory. Pay attention to what feels best to you—sucking, licking, or nibbling. Which is more satisfying? Which is more arousing?*

❖ *The next time you make love, experiment with edible lubricants or with whipped cream, chocolate, or honey. This is especially beneficial to those who are new to oral sex and those who are offended by bodily tastes and smells.*

⑥ Touch ②

With our skin as the medium, our sense of touch provides us with a vital source of information about our close surroundings, our state of being, and our contact with reality and those to whom we are closest. Those who lack sight or hearing rely primarily on their sense of touch to help them explore and experience the world, and they often develop acute sensitivity in their hands. You can also experience this sensitivity by closing your eyes or blindfolding yourself and feeling different textures and shapes, totally immersing yourself in the nuances of sensation. Run your fingers lightly over an object. Is it cold or warm? Is it smooth or rough? Are its edges sharp or blunt?

Touch also provides us with a major source of pleasure, relaxation, healing, and arousal. Of all our senses, touch is the one most central to lovemaking. The feel of your lover's skin can simultaneously excite, reassure, and bond you with your partner.

Our skin is the organ that provides us with the most information. It constantly gives us messages about the environment in which we live. By expanding your awareness of your skin, you can develop your perceptions and thus expand your awareness of the world you live in. Awakening to the sensitivity of your skin can help you become more sensitive to others, especially your lover, and becoming more conscious of your skin and your sense of touch can make you a better lover.

The following exercises will help you to heighten your awareness of your skin and your sense of touch.

1. Take a walk in a park, your neighborhood, or at the beach. Focus your attention on how the air feels on your skin. Be conscious of its temperature and whether or not it is moving. Feel the air on your face, your arms and legs, wherever your skin is bare. Feel the wind in your hair. Take off your shoes and walk across the grass or sand. Feel the textures, how warm or cool the grass or sand is beneath your feet.

2. You can enrich even everyday tasks by focusing on the "feel" of the experience rather than by just doing it mechanically.

For example, the next time you wash your hair, try doing it slowly and deliberately. If you usually race through this task, take your time and slow down instead. Enjoy the feel of the foam on your hands and the sensual rubbing of your hands on your scalp. Notice the sensations on your scalp, your fingertips, and your face.

3. Develop your awareness of your skin by spending a few minutes each day exploring the way it feels on different parts of your body. Start by touching the back of your neck, behind your ears, and the sides of your cheeks. Notice how touching each area makes you feel. Now touch the entire surface of your left hand and arm. Notice any variation in sensitivity between the palm and the back of your hand, the inside and the outside of your arm. Lie down on your back and touch first one side and then the other side of your torso. Notice whether there are any differences in how one side feels versus the other.

4. This is a variation of the sensory basket exercise presented earlier. Once again, select a variety of objects, as different in weight and texture as possible. Your collection might include a shell or stone, a fur glove, an ice cube, a flower, a spoon, a silk scarf, and a feather. Place the objects on a table in front of you. This time, instead of exploring each object using all five senses, close your eyes. Explore each object thoroughly, noticing any differences in texture and temperature. Do you notice more with your eyes closed? How does it make you feel to explore without seeing?

5. Begin to notice the various textures of your life—the cool sheets against your skin, the comforting roughness of towels, the carpet beneath your feet. Imagine how boring your life would be if everything had the same texture. Now focus your attention on the various textures of your body—the softness or coarseness of your hair, the hardness and smoothness of your nails and teeth, the varying degrees of softness and roughness of your skin.

❖ *The next time you and your partner are in bed together, touch your
partner's body as if you were doing so for the first time. Notice the
differences in texture—how some parts of her body are softer than
others. You can do this with your eyes closed if you wish, imagining
you are blind and must get to know her by feel. Notice how some parts
of her body are warmer than others, how some are more enjoyable to
touch. Pay attention to how you feel as you do this exercise, since it
can create a sense of intimacy you may not be used to.*

❖ *Experiment with various types of touch to discover what turns each of
you on or off. Try using your fingernails to lightly scratch his arms, or
use your heel or a knuckle to press deeply into his back. Try lightly
touching the back of his legs, using just your fingertips. Get a little
wild and see how he likes the feel of your hair against his buttocks or
how he likes it when you lick his toes.*

⑥ Using All Your Senses ⑥

It is difficult to experience the beauty and variety the world has to offer if
you are out of touch with your senses. It is also difficult to experience your
partner or your own sensuality fully.

Most of us have the tendency to rely on just one or two of our senses.
For example, we normally rely on our sight to experience an environment
or a person. But just seeing something is not a complete experience of it—
you need to be able to feel it and smell it. You may even need to hear and
taste it. The following exercise will encourage you to explore your environment using all your senses, even those you normally would not focus on
such as taste.

Exercise | **The Blindfold**

Preparation: Do this exercise with your partner. First, each of you select some objects of various textures: ice cubes, a peeled orange, feathers, a silk scarf, flowers. Make sure you don't let your partner see what you've chosen.

1. Decide who will be blindfolded first.

2. The unblindfolded partner will now place each item into the hands, under the feet, against the elbows, or behind the knees of the one who is blindfolded. Each item should be thoroughly explored!

3. Ask the blindfolded person to guess what the item is, turning it into a game if you feel like it (with the prize being something very sexy).

4. Trade places and see who comes up with the most correct answers.

You can play the same game by selecting items with various smells or tastes.

The following exercises will encourage you to open up still further to your senses by exploring the various tastes, smells, sounds, and textures of fruit. The first exercise is to be done alone, the second with your partner.

Exercise | **The Sensuous Orange**

Buy at least one ripe orange, one that is large enough to peel easily. Choose a time and place that will be conducive to a quiet, contemplative experience.

Pick up your orange and look at it closely. Observe its rich color, including any subtle variations. Notice its weight and the cool, curved feeling of its rind against your skin. Slowly roll it around in your hands and feel it yielding to your fingers as you lightly squeeze it.

Now slowly begin peeling the orange. Notice the feeling of your fingertips piercing the rind and pulling it away from the inner fruit. Listen to the sound of the skin being pulled apart, and notice the sharp aroma of the oil as it drifts from the rind into the air. Smell the aroma growing stronger as you hold the orange closer to your face.

Pull apart the inner sections and spread the entire fruit open in your hands. Feel the wetness of the orange, smell the milder aroma of its juice, and observe the way the light reflects on its translucent surfaces.

Finally, completely pull apart the orange and put one section in your mouth. Feel its soft wetness on your lips and tongue, then gently bite it and feel the fresh orange juice squirting into your mouth. Feel the texture of the orange on the inside of your mouth. Chew the orange until you have extracted the sweet, pungent juices and flavors. Swallow and feel the orange moving down your throat. As you consume the rest of the orange, continue paying full attention to all your senses in the same way.

E x e r c i s e | **The Sensuous Fruit Fest**

This exercise is a variation of the Tom Jones Dinner developed in the 1970s, based on the novel by Henry Fielding (and the movie based on the novel) in which a couple seduces each other with food. During this exercise, some people spontaneously begin taking food from each other's mouths, others rub the fruit on each other's bodies and then lick off the juices. [3]

1. Go to the market and pick out a variety of sensuous fruits. Figs, strawberries, and mangos make good candidates. Spend as much time as necessary choosing the juiciest, most pungent, most erotic fruit you can find to share with each other.

2. Choose an environment in which you can be alone and undisturbed for a long time. If you choose to do this exercise outside, find a secluded place where you will not be disturbed by passersby.

3. Spread a large plastic tablecloth or drop cloth on the ground or on your floor at home. Wash your hands, and then spread all the fruit out in front of you. Make sure you are wearing clothes that you won't mind staining, or, better yet, do this exercise in the nude.

4. Begin exploring the various fruits, paying attention to the different ways they smell, sound, and feel in your hands. Pick up a piece of fruit that looks especially tempting, one that you would like to share with your partner. Slowly, very slowly, bite into it. Keeping your eyes on each other, savor each flavor as it spreads over your tongue. Now seductively, teasingly, offer a bite to your partner.

5. Continue to feed each other ripe bananas, juicy oranges, stimulating kiwi, velvety mango and papaya, and succulent, sensuous strawberries. Don't be shy about sharing the fruit in other more daring ways.

To reconnect with your natural sensuality, continue giving yourself permission to explore all your senses. You can explore in whatever ways are comfortable and natural for you. If you are artistic you may do so by allowing yourself to experiment with clay or finger paints. If you are athletic you can explore by connecting more with your body, noticing how it feels as you run through the air or swim through the water. If you are a nature buff, you can explore by appreciating nature—the sweet smell of new-mowed grass and flowers, the crunch of sand under your feet, the chirping of the morning birds.

Once you have begun to open up to your senses you will undoubtedly feel more connected to your body. You will find that your vitality is increased and your perceptions are heightened. You will feel more sensitive to both your own and your partner's needs. You may discover that you are also beginning to feel more sensual and possibly more sexual. Those of you who have been suffering from a lack of sexual desire may begin to feel the juices flowing again, and those of you who have felt distant from your partner, for whatever reason, may feel slightly more open to her. You may even begin to notice that some of the feelings you felt when you first fell in love may begin to re-emerge.

The exercises in the following chapter will open you still further to the many sensual possibilities that lie ahead for you and will offer you still more opportunities to connect with your partner in a sensuously erotic way.

. . . .

Let me apply the unguent

of aloe leaves

let me rub

your feet which brought you to this shack

by the sea.

You lie beneath the Indian

scarves and shawls

away from the freeway and the overpass.

Join the secret rites

join the kiva.

The dunes are spilling over with ice plant.

Between us

all is sacred

heal

my love.

— FROM "INVITATION TO THE KIVA,"
BY GLENNA LUSCHEI

CHAPTER FOUR

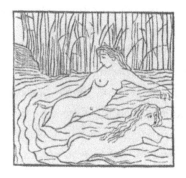

Liquid Love

S tress can cause couples to become critical of and short-tempered with each other or distant and disinterested. It can erode love, chipping away at it until there is little left of the warmth, excitement, and intimacy you once felt for each other.

Controlling stress, separately and together, is an important step toward engaging in Sensual Sex. Today more than ever we all need to learn more effective ways to relax and to make relaxation a part of our sexual relationships. Because stress has become such a large part of our lives, we need to learn ways to reconnect with our bodies and with our partner as well as with the beauty and tranquillity of life.

In this chapter you will learn sensuous ways to relax, techniques that will encourage you to connect with each other in a relaxed, unstressful way. Since being relaxed is a key to sexual pleasure, this is a significant chapter. I have entitled it "Liquid Love" because in it you will learn techniques that will help dissolve the tension, wash away the worries of the outside world, and lower your defenses so you can melt into each other's arms.

We will begin by focusing on the many healing benefits of water and on water as an avenue for awakening feelings of sensuality and sexuality. Exploring the sensuality of water can be especially healing, because we all have deep connections with and strong memories of water that for most of us are overwhelmingly positive. Therefore, exploring your body and your partner's in the water can make the experience feel more comfortable and less threatening than it might be otherwise.

⑤ Water As Liquid Love ⑥

Most of us have an inborn instinct about how to use water to reduce stress. We somehow know that we can find sedation and comfort in a warm bath and stimulus in a short, cold shower.

Water, especially warm water, is essentially relaxing. It relaxes our muscles, soothes our nerves, and calms our emotions. Some scientists say that we feel better in water because the sea is our true ancestral home.

Others liken the feeling of relaxation in water to the memory of the amniotic fluid in which we were suspended before birth.

Water is the most sensual of all the elements, and some of our most intensely sensuous experiences are associated with it. Playing in the sprinkler on a hot summer's day. Sinking into a pool of water on a moonlit night. Canoeing on a lake with a lover, stopping under some trees to make love. Becoming mesmerized as the sun sets over the water. Tasting the salt and feeling the crisp sea breeze as you glide effortlessly over the waves in a sailboat. The smell of the ocean, the sound of the waves crashing against the shore, the way the sun makes it shimmer and shine—all these images evoke strong sense memories, often of romantic interludes or other times of joy and peace.

Water has long been the friend of lovers. In novels and films we witness couples running through the rain together, stopping to embrace and kiss, drops of water glistening on their skin or lovers locked in a passionate embrace, rolling on the sand, the ocean waves washing over them.

Water evokes not only a feeling of sensuality and sexuality but also one of freedom. We often feel less inhibited when we're in or near the water. Buoyed up by the water, we often feel lighter, more playful and energized. Warm water in particular evokes feelings of comfort and security. It reminds us of our childhood baths—the caressing water, being stroked and soothed by the hands of those who cared for us—and we began to associate these pleasant sensations with mother and love and safety.

Water is a natural medicine that benefits the entire body. Water therapy, or hydrotherapy, originated in ancient times and is used in a variety of versatile ways to treat many medical and psychological conditions. We know from fragments of medical history that the eminent Greek physician Hippocrates advocated the medicinal use of baths. One of the early and great clinical observers, he noted a direct correlation between the use of partial and full baths and the healing of many diseases. A remarkable reenergizer, water therapy restores the energy flow, helps the body to heal itself, and prevents other health problems from occurring.

In many cultures, water also represents healing, purification, renewal, and rebirth. For this reason water has been used throughout history in religious and other rituals to represent cleansing of the body and spirit.

The Bath

Taking a bath is fast becoming one of the most popular ways to reduce stress, relax tired muscles, and rejuvenate the spirit. Bath oils, bath salts, and essential oils are all becoming popular as we reinvent the bath to meet our modern needs.

Many ancient cultures used baths for ritual and health purposes, to maximize beauty, promote alertness, and eliminate stress. Chambers built specifically for the bath may have been created by the Egyptians. Bathing was also an integral ritual in Jewish tribal life. Even in the Middle Ages, when the Church frowned on bathing, the Jews maintained public bath houses. The ancient Minoans left the remnants of bathing apartments in the palaces of Cnossus and Tiryns, as did the ancient Greeks, who created luxurious bathing areas complete with heated water, cold showers, and plunging pools.

You can vary your bath, depending on your mood and needs. Hot baths relax and soothe the body and help you to overcome aches and pains. If you want to ease pain, relax before going to sleep, or to produce perspiration to eliminate toxins, bacteria, or disease from the body, warm or hot baths are most effective. However, long hot baths can deplete your energy and body tone. Cold water, on the other hand, restores body tone. For tonic effects, there is nothing better than cold water. Therefore, no matter what your bathing preference, remember to end each bath or shower with cool or cold water.

The Sensuous Bath

In our fast-paced, stressful world, we rarely allow ourselves the luxury of a full, relaxing bath, and yet a bath can be the most healing and rejuvenating of experiences. By taking just a little extra time out during your day, you can create your own peaceful escape, a place where you can indulge your senses and nurture your soul.

Later in this chapter I provide information on how to create your own personal spa using essential oils, and include more information on hydrotherapy. Just taking a bath can be completely relaxing and rejuvenating, in itself, but once you learn how to incorporate the use of aromatherapy with the basics of hydrotherapy techniques, you'll multiply the bath's effects.

E x e r c i s e | **The Awakening Your Senses Personal Bath**

This exercise will encourage you to continue reconnecting with and exploring your senses and will help you discover more about your body. It is an ideal way to prepare yourself for a romantic interlude with your partner, even if he is not yet enthusiastic about getting involved in the Awakening Your Senses Program.

Preparation: Choose a mild liquid soap with a pleasing smell, plenty of warm, fluffy, luxurious towels to drape yourself in afterwards, a washcloth or bathing sponge, candles, and soothing or erotic music or recorded nature sounds. As you fill your tub with warm water (add bath oil or bubble bath if desired), light some candles and place them close to the tub and turn on your music (very low so it won't be too distracting). Make sure the room is warm enough and that your towels are within reach.

Roll up one of the towels to use as a headrest while you luxuriate in the warm, but not too hot, water. Slowly immerse yourself in the water. As you do, pay attention to how it feels on your skin. Notice how the water embraces you, how the moisture makes your skin glisten. Lie back and enjoy your bath for a few moments, clearing your mind of all worries and preoccupations.

Squeeze some liquid soap into the palm of your hand and begin to apply it to your feet. Notice how the cool soap feels against skin that has been warmed by the bath. Apply the soap the way you would apply massage oil, slowly and lovingly spreading it over your feet. As you spread the soap between each toe, notice how sensuous your toes can feel.

Slowly continue applying the soap up your calves to your thighs, making sure you spend lots of time caressing your knees. For many people, women especially, the front and back of the knees are especially sensitive and can evoke erotic feelings. As you move up your thighs, notice how sensitive the inside of your thighs can be, especially as you move closer and closer to your genitals.

Now begin to soap your genitals, but do so in a slower, less perfunctory way than you would normally, paying attention to how the soap feels against your skin, using the soap to explore all the nooks and crannies. If you become aroused, great! Don't stop now to masturbate, but continue up your body to complete the exercise.

Gently apply soap to your stomach, and continue spreading it out over your entire torso as far as you can reach, including the often neglected sides of your body.

Notice which part of your torso is most sensitive to the touch— your stomach, your chest, or the sides of your body. If you're a woman, spend extra time applying soap to your breasts. Make sure you lift each breast and apply soap underneath and that you include the sides of your breasts and under your arms. Which part of your breasts is most sensitive to the touch? Take time to apply soap to your nipples, allowing yourself to become aroused as you do so.

Now apply soap to your arms, starting at the top and working your way down with long, continuous strokes. Notice how good it feels as you smooth the soap onto the inside of your arms, especially around the elbow. Take time to slather the soap onto your hands, the inside of your wrists, and your forearms and notice how good it feels when you smooth it over these areas.

Smooth soap over your neck and shoulders, reaching as far back as you can to include as much of your back as possible. Notice how sensitive the sides of your neck and the tops of your shoulders can be. Experiment by lightly tickling these areas with your fingertips.

Finally, lie back, place a small amount of soap on your fingertips, and begin to apply it to your face and the outside of your ears. (If you don't wish to have soap on your face, cup some water in your hand and follow the same instructions.) Gently touch each part of your face, noticing which places are most sensitive (around your mouth? the sides of your cheeks? your forehead?). Now spend time exploring your ears, including the backs of your earlobes. Once again, use your fingertips to slightly tickle different areas on your face and ears and notice the delicate sensations that this elicits.

After your bath, pat (don't rub) your skin dry with a warm, clean towel and lovingly massage some lotion into your skin. Notice how relaxed and how much more connected to your body you feel.

Self-Healing Rituals

In addition to helping you connect with your body and your sensuality, bathing can also help heal you of physical discomfort, stress, and emotional wounds. By combining bathing with self-healing rituals, you can gain a sense of being reborn, cleansed, and refreshed. People who suffer from a poor body image, who have been physically, sexually, or emotionally violated, or who suffer from shame associated with their body can also benefit from self-healing rituals.

Exercise | **A Cleansing Ritual**

As you soak yourself in a hot bath or Jacuzzi, let the water rinse away fatigue and tension. Allow the weight of the world and all the stress you carry around with you to float away on the water. Imagine that all the residues of your stressful life are being soaked out of you through your skin. Visualize the impurities flowing out of your pores.

If you experience physical discomfort or pain, visualize the water diluting the pain, or imagine the healing water bringing health to your body. If you have been physically or sexually abused, imagine impurities flowing out of your genitals, breasts, anus, or any place that feels contaminated by the abuse.

Now imagine love pouring into your body, restoring you to optimum health. Visualize yourself being reborn into a body that is pure and healthy. Emerge from the water cleansed, inside and out.

Exercise | **The Opening Your Heart Ritual**

As you soak in the warm water, imagine that you are being enveloped by an ocean of love. Visualize your heart opening up to the love and warmth that is all around you. Know that you are a caring human being, worthy of being loved and cherished. Let the water wash away all the barriers keeping you from loving yourself, from loving others, and from allowing others to love you.

By inventing your own personal ritual, you can reclaim your body for your own sensual and sexual enjoyment. Your ritual can be combined with a series of positive affirmations such as, "My body is healthy and strong. As I learn to take better care of it, it will continue to take care of my needs" or "I deserve to love and to be loved."

Continue to turn everyday bathing into an act dedicated to honoring and respecting your body, and continue to practice bathing rituals to purify yourself and to energize your body. By loving your body in this way you empower yourself and increase your self-esteem.

Shared Bathing Experiences

As you have discovered after experiencing the Awakening Your Senses Personal Bath, there is no better way to reconnect with oneself and one's sensuality and sexuality than through the luxuriousness of a bath. And what better way to get to know a new lover or to renew the bonds of love with an old one than by experiencing a bath, Jacuzzi, or shower together?

E x e r c i s e | **The Shared Sensuous Bath**

Preparation: You'll need candles, romantic or erotic music, liquid soap, and several large, luxurious towels. Help set the mood by removing everyday items such as toothbrushes, cosmetics, or children's toys.

You can either face each other in the tub with your legs wrapped around each other or sit front to back, one of you leaning against the tub with your legs surrounding your partner and the other leaning against your partner's chest.

If you can't both fit in the tub, you can take turns, with one of you sitting on the rim of the tub while the other soaks.

In this exercise you will follow the instructions for the personal bath described above, with these exceptions. Instead of applying liquid soap to your own body, you will apply it to your partner's body. Obviously, you will not have the same access to your partner's body as you did to your own, but you can easily reach her feet, legs, thighs, chest and arms, shoulders, and face. If you huddle together you can even reach each other's backs! Your partner's stomach and genitals may be harder to reach depending on your respective body sizes.

To begin, one person should be the passive receiver and the other the active giver. Both giver and receiver should keep talking to a minimum— only talk if something feels uncomfortable or especially delightful.

When you are the active giver focus all your attention on how your partner's body feels to the touch—its curves, how different the smooth areas feel from the rough areas, and so on. Focus on how it feels to you as you gently, slowly smooth the soap over her body. Do not ask your partner how it feels; just assume it feels wonderful unless you hear otherwise. As you stroke, feel the sensations of your skin sliding over your lover's flesh.

When you are the passive receiver focus all your attention on how your skin feels being caressed with the soap. Don't worry about your partner and whether he is getting tired or bored or feels cramped in the tub. Don't direct your partner in how he could do it better. Lie back and let yourself be swept away by the sensations being bestowed upon you as you're lulled by the warmth of the water.

When you get out of the tub, take turns drying off each other's bodies. Don't rub, softly pat. Drying each other off can feel like a very comforting, caring gesture. Take your time and make sure you dry off your partner's entire body.

E x e r c i s e | **The Shared Sensual Shower**

You've no doubt had the experience of showering with a lover. Some people love to shower together, soaping each other, splashing water in each other's faces, holding each other's wet, slippery bodies, often culminating in lovemaking. Sadly, most couples discontinue this sensual treat after the newness of the relationship wears off.

In this exercise you will be reintroduced to the shared shower and possibly learn some new variations on soaping and caressing.

Preparation: Choose a mild, liquid soap, a bathing sponge, at least two luxurious towels, and candles if you wish to shower in a semidarkened room. Know ahead of time that you are going to get your hair wet, that you will no doubt use all the hot water, and that you are going to spend at least a half-hour in the shower.

As with the bathing exercise above, when you are the receiver, your focus should be on relaxing and enjoying the touches, not on how your partner is feeling. The only time you should speak is when something feels uncomfortable or especially pleasurable, but do avoid directing your partner's movements.

Take turns applying plenty of liquid soap onto each other's bodies, starting with the shoulders, back, buttocks, and the backs of each other's legs (you can forego the feet, since it will be difficult and possibly dangerous for your partner to balance on one foot). Apply the soap gently and slowly instead of rubbing it on. Linger over each sensuous inch of your lover's body. Explore each groove and curve. Try using the flat of your hand, the back of your wrist, and your forearm to spread the soap. Really get into it. Find areas of your partner's body that feel especially good to touch, and spend extra time there.

Now proceed to the front of your partner's body, taking care to make sure his face is not directly under the flow of the shower faucet. Skip his face and start with the shoulders, chest, arms, and stomach. Then move down to the pelvic area, the genitals, and finally the thighs and calves. Once again, focus on how it feels to you to touch your lover's skin in this way and concentrate on finding areas that feel especially sensuous to you.

Apply more soap on both of you, and standing back to front begin rubbing your bodies together in a sensuous dance. Slide your hands up and down your slippery bodies. Turn front to front and continue your dance, letting your hands and bodies sculpture each curve of each other's bodies. What you do from here on is up to you.

You can choose to rinse off after each person's turn or remain soaped up for the finale. (You will want to rinse off your genitals, however, as even the mildest soap can irritate delicate membranes.)

To complete your sensuous interlude, rinse your lover with soothing streams of water from the sponge. Then dry each other off with soft towels, patting rather than rubbing.

Exercise | **The Foot Bath and Caress**

This is another wonderful exercise to do with your partner. It is a deeply relaxing, sensuous experience that can help each of you to get out of your heads and to focus on your body and on your senses. Because this exercise is nonthreatening, it is also a good one for couples who feel a lot of pressure to perform.

Preparation: You'll need two towels, a basin or tub large enough for a person's feet, liquid soap, warm water, and oil or lotion. The passive person will need to sit in a chair with his or her feet on the floor. Since this exercise includes the ankles and part of the calves, the passive partner should either wear shorts or loose, comfortable pants that can be easily rolled up. The entire experience should take approximately one hour.

E x e r c i s e | When You Are the Active Partner

Fill the basin with warm water and place your partner's feet in the water. If you do not have a basin large enough for both feet, do one foot at a time. Place some liquid soap in the palm of your hand and slowly caress your partner's feet, ankles, and lower calves. Remember to touch for your own pleasure, caressing the skin as opposed to massaging muscles. Bathe one foot at a time, finding out how the different areas of the foot feel as you bathe them. Use not only your fingers but your palm, wrist, and forearm to caress and smooth the soap onto your partner's body. When you discover an area of the foot, ankle, or lower calf that feels especially sensuous to you, spend extra time there, enjoying the feeling. You can gently lift each foot out of the water and cradle it in your free hand if you'd like. This provides the opportunity for you to caress the arch and the bottom of the foot (this usually works only when your partner's foot is rather small and light). Spend at least five minutes on each foot, but take longer if you'd like.

When you are finished with both feet, lift each foot out of the water firmly but gently, dry them, and wrap them in separate towels. Put aside the basin. Now gently take one foot from the towel and caress it, using the oil or lotion. Take as long as you like, staying longer on parts of the foot, ankle, and lower calf that you especially enjoy touching. Spend at least five to ten minutes on each foot.

Always maintain contact with your partner as you are giving the caress to avoid surprising her with a sudden touch when you switch hands. If you use lotion or oil, warm it in your hand before you apply it, and maintain contact with your partner's body when you reapply the lotion.

Make sure that you are going very, very slowly; the slower the better. If you think you are moving your hand slowly enough, cut your speed in half and see how this affects your ability to focus on the touch. Don't worry about whether your partner is enjoying the caress. It will be her responsibility to let you know if you are doing something that makes her feel uncomfortable.

While it is normal to become distracted now and then, if you find your mind wandering, try bringing it back to the place where your skin makes contact with your partner's.

Do not speak while doing the exercise and do not ask for feedback. Assume that your caresses feel good, or at least neutral.

Exercise | When You Are the Passive Partner

To start, the passive person sits in a chair with her feet on the floor. If you aren't wearing shorts, roll your pant legs up.

As the passive person during the foot bath and caress, all you need do is relax, enjoy, and allow yourself to be pampered. If your partner does something that bothers you, say something, but otherwise concentrate completely on his touch. Relax your feet and let them just hang from your legs. Your partner will lift them into the basin and move them—you don't need to help.

Close your eyes and try to relax any muscles that feel tense. Keep your attention on the place where your partner is touching your skin. Mentally follow his hand as it caresses your body. Do not give your partner any feedback unless something feels painful or uncomfortable. Do not moan or groan or wiggle around, because this can be a subtle way of manipulating the active partner into continuing to touch a particular spot. Remaining completely passive will allow you to experience pleasure more fully. If you become tense, try taking some deep breaths to relax yourself, and focus only on the touch.

Feedback

At the end of the exercise, talk openly and honestly with each other about your experience. You will not get the full benefit from the exercise if you lie about your feelings. For instance, please do not tell your partner you enjoyed the experience if you didn't or that you were able to concentrate if you weren't, just so you appear to be doing things correctly.

Most people benefit greatly from giving and receiving feedback after the exercises. This kind of feedback can be the beginning of honest communication and the establishment of trust and openness. Most learn to communicate more openly and honestly about what feels good and what doesn't, and they also learn what feels good to their partner.

Sensual Massage and Essential Oils as Liquid Love

In this section we'll discuss another form of liquid love—massage and essential oils. Nothing feels more loving than to have your partner anoint your body with warm, sensuous oil. And essential oils can act as an aphrodisiac—stirring feelings of longing and desire in even the most stressed-out, indifferent lover.

The therapeutic use of oils dates back thousands of years to the ancient Egyptians, Indians, and Chinese. Egypt's climate was then, as it is now, hot, dusty and dry, and it had a devastating effect on people's skins. Servants of the very rich massaged perfumed oils into the skins of their masters to stop dryness and to maintain the suppleness and sensuality of youth. Pregnant women had special oil-based unguents that they massaged into their skins to prevent stretch marks.

The Greeks learned from the Egyptians and used essential oils in their baths and massages. Hippocrates prescribed aromatic baths and scented massage oils for protection against contagious diseases.

In addition to scented baths and massages, the Romans rubbed scented oils on the feet of their guests at banquets. In the Middle Ages, monks cultivated herbs and discovered many of their restorative properties. Among the first to distill plant essences, they carefully blended them into liqueurs to be administered to patients.

Oiling

Most people haven't been gently oiled by another person since early child-hood when it was an exquisitely tender experience, usually shared between parent and child. Whether or not you combine it with massage or caressing, oiling your partner's body can be extremely pleasurable for both of you, helping you to relax and to reconnect emotionally as well as physically.

Moreover, oiling your partner's body makes nearly every massage movement easier. Oil allows your hands to move smoothly without pulling at the skin and adds not only to your partner's pleasure but to your own.

When selecting an oil be aware that any high-quality, cold-pressed vegetable oil like safflower and sesame seed will work as well as the high-priced commercial products. Coconut oil is ideal for massage, since it liquefies at room temperature, but olive and peanut oil are too thick. Many people recommend that you not use petroleum-based oils, since they are considered health risks and because they tend to stain sheets and towels. Some people prefer high-quality water-dispersible massage oils, which do not stain sheets and clothing and are easily rinsed off.

You can scent your oil with a few drops of lemon juice, your partner's favorite scent, or an essential oil (discussed in detail later on in the chapter). Or visit a shop together that sells massage oils and pick one that has a scent you both find enjoyable.

An excellent way to improve any massage experience is to warm your massage oil by placing it in a pan of hot water. The warm oil will feel exquisite on your lover's skin, warming his heart and heating up his passion. Keep your oil in a small plastic squeeze bottle to prevent spills. Never pour oil directly onto your partner's body; instead, pour it first into your hands. To maintain contact, press the back of your hand or fingers against your partner's body while you pour oil into your palms. The temperature of your hands should also warm the oil, and if it feels cool, rub your hands together to warm it.

Apply just enough oil so that you can still feel your partner's skin as your hands glide over it. Whenever you feel your partner's skin drying out, add more oil. Avoid using too much, because doing so will cause your hands to skid over your partner's body. Don't confuse caress oiling with applying suntan lotion, which is generally rubbed onto the body impersonally. Apply the oil with loving care.

⑥ Essential Oils and Aromatherapy ⑥

An essential oil is a highly concentrated extract from parts of plants such as leaves, stems, bark, flowers, roots, and fruits. The "essence" of a particular plant form, they are responsible for giving a botanical its unique scent and healing properties. For example, when you sniff a rose or a sage bush while taking a walk, you experience the essential oils they release into the air.

Although called "oils," essential oils aren't oily at all but more a water-like fluid. They are volatile, meaning they turn very readily from a liquid to a gas at room temperature or higher. Rupturing the essential oil glands, or heat exposure, also helps release these natural scents. These oils are so potent that one drop of essential oil equals approximately thirty cups of herbal tea in strength.

Technically, *aromatherapy* means simply the "study of scent," but aromatherapy is more thoroughly defined as the skilled and controlled use of essential oils to enhance physical and emotional health and well-being. Practitioners define aromatherapy as the therapeutic use of essential oils to help balance the mind and body.

Today scientific studies are finally confirming what has been known for centuries, that essential oils have healing properties on both physical and emotional levels.

How Essential Oils Enter the Body

Essential oils penetrate the body in two ways, through the nose and through the skin. Again according to Cooksley,

> *the olfactory system, the nose-brain association, is the most direct connection*
> *we have with the environment. Think about how sensitive our sense of smell*
> *is—approximately 10,000 times more sensitive than any other sensory organ*
> *we possess. The fact that our sense of smell is linked directly to the limbic brain*
> *where emotions, memory, and certain regulatory functions are seated makes me*
> *realize how this important route of absorption is neglected in everyday life.* [4]

According to Cooksley, there are several variables involved in using the nose as a point of entry. Obviously, the most significant factor is how keen one's sense of smell is. If a person smokes, this will undoubtedly affect his ability to smell, and some head injuries or a stroke can also cause dysfunction in this area. Age can be a factor (our ability to smell is at its peak between the ages of twenty and forty), as can the time of day, with nighttime being when we are most sensitive. Women have the greatest acuity when scent is involved, especially when they are ovulating.

The second way for essential oils to enter the body is through the skin, which is a two-way structure designed to keep some things in and others out. Our pores allow the free passage into our body of the things we need, and the passage of waste products out.

Because essential oils are organic and have an inherently low molecular weight, they are absorbed through the pores and hair follicles of the skin. The time interval for absorption will vary depending on the condition of the skin. Poor circulation, thick toughened skin, or excessive cellulite or fat may slow down the rate of absorption, whereas heat, water, broken or damaged skin, or exercise will cause increased absorption. Finally, the carrier or base used may affect the absorption rate, since some vegetable oils are heavier than others.

The following is a listing of popular base or carrier oils.

* ❖ *Good for all skin types: safflower, sunflower, sweet almond*
* ❖ *Good for dry skin types: avocado, evening primrose*
* ❖ *Good for oily skin types: hazelnut*
* ❖ *Good for mature or sensitive skin: peach or apricot kernel oil*
* ❖ *Best when mixed with other carrier oils: olive, vitamin E, wheat germ, avocado, evening primrose*

You may wish to have at least two of these base carriers on hand, since they have different consistencies and can be used for different purposes.

Essential oils are very strong and therefore should never be applied to the skin undiluted. Even diluted, some oils may cause an allergic reaction in some people, so it is best to do a patch test before using them. Some oils such as basil, clary sage, cedarwood, hyssop, ginger, marjoram, sage, pennyroyal, and thyme should not be used by pregnant women. If you are prone to allergic reactions, are pregnant, or suffer from high blood pressure, epilepsy, or other neural disorders, you should consult a medical practitioner or professional aromatherapist before using aromatherapy.

The proportion of essential oil to base carrier or water is very important. Use only small amounts of essential oil; the recommended proportions of essential oils to base carrier oils are twelve drops of oil to five teaspoons of carrier. Pregnant women should use even less oil.

Aromatic Baths

Bathing with essential oils, or aromatic bathing, will help you transform your bath into a personal spa, which will provide not only an incredibly sensuous experience but also deep relaxation, rejuvenation, and healing. As stated earlier, every essential oil has the potential to affect us both physically and emotionally. Since the molecular structure of essential oils enables them to easily penetrate the skin, essential oils used in the bath can be particularly effective. In addition to their ability to heal the body, they also affect our moods, since we inhale them as they evaporate.

Carriers, such as oil blends, are needed to disperse the essential oils in the bath, since the oils are not soluble in water. Some popular carrier agents—canola, soy, safflower, and sweet almond oils—are wonderful moisturizers but can also leave an oily ring in the bathtub. To avoid this you can use carriers such as honey, Castile soap, sweet cream, or a "bath salt" mixture instead. (Bath salts have the added benefit of being great detoxifying and "drawing-out" agents.)

When using essential oils without a carrier, always add them after the tub has been filled, because they evaporate very quickly. Give them a swish in the water with your hand to ensure that they disperse as much as possible.

For a full soak make sure your shoulders are completely submerged. It is generally recommended that you spend from twenty to thirty minutes in the bath to get the full benefit.

Here are some suggestions for various types of baths:

❖ *For a soothing bath, mix five to ten drops of essential oil in 1/4 cup of raw honey, than add to bath water.*

❖ *For a healing bath, add one or two vitamin E capsules by cutting off the end of a gel cap and squeezing the vitamin E oil into the honey, mixing well.*

❖ *To soften dry skin, add five to ten drops of essential oil to 1/4 to 1/2 cup of heavy cream, buttermilk, or goat's milk and add to bath.*

❖ *To replenish and nourish the entire body, add five to ten drops of essential oil to 1/4 cup of aloe vera or juice.*

❖ *To detoxify the body, add five to ten drops of essential oil to one teaspoon of baking soda, two teaspoons of Epsom salt, and three teaspoons of sea salt. Mix well. Add to bath water.*

Lavender oil is highly recommended since it has been used for centuries to heal various skin conditions and for skin rejuvenation, as well as for soothing the nervous system.

Stimulating Showers

If you prefer showers to baths, you can still enjoy the benefits of aromatherapy. Before getting into the shower, massage yourself with a cloth sprinkled with six to eight drops of essential oils and then shower as usual. Your pores will be opened by the heat from the water, allowing some of the oils to be absorbed and diffusing aromatic scents around you. Keep the bathroom door shut to keep in the vapor. (This massage method is not recommended for sensitive areas or on broken or irritated skin. Also, do not use peppermint essential oil undiluted on the skin or other skin-irritant essential oils such as aniseed, basil, bay, benzoin, camphor, citronella, fennel, lemongrass, lemon verbena, rose, rosemary, or ylang-ylang.)

A second way of using essential oils in the shower is to apply them after you have washed but before you get out. Put your essential oils on your wet washcloth and rub yourself all over, breathing deeply as the water runs down your body. Once you are out of the shower, gently towel off, taking care not to scrub off all the good oils you just put on.

A third option is the "ministeambath method." Plug the shower drain (a rubber stopper works especially well) and add a few drops of essential oils to the water collecting in the bottom of the shower. This way you will be inhaling the beneficial steam as the vapors rise as well as soaking your feet in the aromatic water collecting in the tub.

Essential Oils Known to Be Aphrodisiacs

Aphrodisiacs—substances capable of enhancing sexual pleasure or sexual desire—have been around for a long time. Throughout the ages various foods have been used to energize the body and to affect circulation, which in turn often produces a positive effect on the entire body—including the sexual organs—and the emotions. Traditional herbs have also been used for centuries to stimulate circulation and to aid in conditions such as erectile dysfunction. Finally, perfume was used to influence the emotions directly and as a personal scent to attract romance and love.

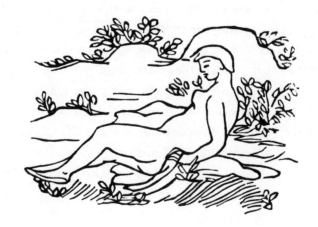

More than those present in perfume, the essential oils used in aromotherapy have the potential to affect the circulatory, hormonal, and nervous systems. Essential oils are mood-enhancing substances capable of creating, for example, warmth, euphoria, romance, or spirituality.

Aphrodisiacs can also be used to enhance feelings of self-confidence, joy, and a general feeling of well-being. Aromatherapy is thought to have unlimited potential in this area. According to Cooksley,

> *the olfactory system and its direct association with the limbic system is real and powerful. Pleasure, reproductive cycles, sex drive, memory, and emotions are seated in the limbic brain. The therapeutic application of essential oils can ease stress and promote relaxation, which can in turn aid with 'performance' issues."* [5]

Patchouli, ginger, and myrrh are especially useful in helping us let go of the worries of the world and become more aware of our bodies.

Earlier, we discussed the important role our olfactory system plays in our sexual functioning. Sometimes a decreased interest in sex is caused by an underactive pituitary gland. The pituitary, also known as the master gland of the endocrine system, is responsible for controlling hormone production of other glands. Essential oils have the ability to stimulate the pituitary gland, and interestingly, consist of many of the essences known to be aphrodisiacs—clary sage, jasmine, patchouli, and ylang-ylang.

The best aphrodisiacs make use of the brain, where the sexual center is located. By incorporating essential oils into your lovemaking, you can create a romantic retreat and escape into a state of mind unlike anything you've ever experienced. Essential oils that have aphrodisiac properties are carrot seed, clary sage, black pepper, ginger, fennel, frankincense, geranium, hyssop, jasmine, juniper, myrrh, neroli, patchouli, pine, rose, rosemary, sandalwood, and ylang-ylang.

Care needs to be taken, however, when you create a scent. Minute and diluted forms of scents must be created with sensitivity. If the blend is too concentrated it will be unpleasant or repulsive rather than erotic. The aim is to create a subtle body odor along with other pleasurable scents that will delight and arouse. Cooksley recommends a blend of the erogenous, stimulating, or calming oils and euphoric essential oils to create a well-rounded aphrodisiac.

Jasmine absolute (which means it was solvent extracted due to its low essential oil content) is the most sought-after fragrance in the perfume industry because it has a very erogenous effect on humans, as does ambrette seed and angelica, which resemble the musk scent.

Aromatherapy applications can be very effective in setting a mood, affecting the emotions, and stimulating the brain to achieve aphrodisia. Aromatic baths, massage oils, and inhalation are most effective because they also encourage intimacy and touch. Essential oils can also be used in the Jacuzzi, sauna, or shower. You can also experiment with sprinkling a few drops onto the bed sheets and using candles, diffusers, and room sprays.

Here are two bath recipes that have aphrodisiac qualities, both inspired by Cooksley's book.

LOVE POTION BATH

1 drop sandalwood
2 drops clary sage
3 drops ylang-ylang

Light candles and place them all around the bathroom and around the edges of the bath. Red candles are particularly effective. Play some intense, exotic music or classical music.

NOSTALGIA BATH *(particularly effective for baby boomers)*

3 drops patchouli

4 drops ylang-ylang

In addition to lighting some candles (the more exotic the better), burn some patchouli incense and play some sixties music (Janice Joplin, the Mamas and the Papas, Simon and Garfunkel). If you have a lava lamp, bring it into the bathroom too!

Here's a bath that is wonderful in the summer or whenever you want to feel like you're on a romantic tropical holiday.

TROPICAL PARADISE BATH

8 drops gardenia oil

8 drops oil of amber

1 ten-ounce can of unsweetened coconut milk

Fill the room with plants and tropical flowers, open the bathroom window, and hang wind chimes. Slice pineapple, papaya, and mango to feed to each other while you are in the tub and imagine yourselves in a tropical paradise. (Rub papaya and mango on your skin for a tantalizing sensation.)

Aromatherapy Massage

Below is a very sensual massage oil designed for the entire body (2 percent dilution), again inspired by Cooksley's book. In order to increase absorption, Valerie suggests you warm the oil in a hot-water bath before you apply it. If the oil seems too strongly scented, simply add more vegetable oil to dilute it further. This makes enough for two people.

LOVER'S OIL

4 tablespoons sweet almond or safflower oil
10 drops sandalwood essential oil
4 drops clary sage essential oil
6 drops ylang-ylang essential oil

Mix the essential oils with warm safflower or sweet almond oil in a shallow dish. Apply to the body in small amounts using a comfortable pressure and working toward the heart. Avoid the face and the genital area.

And here's a recipe for my favorite aphrodisiac massage oil:

6 ounces of any vegetable oil
10 drops jasmine essential oil
10 drops mandarin essential oil
5 drops nutmeg essential oil

For more information on essential oils, including how and where to purchase and store them, please refer to the Resources and Recommended Reading sections in the back of the book.

We have seen how the sensuousness of warm water and massage or essential oils can truly feel like liquid love when shared with someone you care deeply about. You've learned how immersing yourself in the water's peacefulness and savoring the water's warmth can help you get more in touch with your own and your partner's body and prepare you for wonderful lovemaking. Continue to let the sensuousness of water melt away your tension and allow your cares to float away. Cradle and nurture your lover in this watery cocoon as you are reborn together. Feel yourself enveloped by an ocean of love and nourishment for your body and soul, infusing you both with new warmth and vitality.

Smooth oil, like liquid gold, over your lover's body. Watch for the special smile that signals the release of her tension. Listen carefully to hear your lover's blissful moans. Add an aphrodisiac to your oil to broaden the range of sensations and amplify feelings of arousal.

It is better to give and receive.

— Bernard Gunther

Good lovers have known for centuries that the hand is probably the primary sex organ.

— Eleanor Hamilton

Be in your fingers and hands as if your whole being, your whole soul, is there.

— Osho

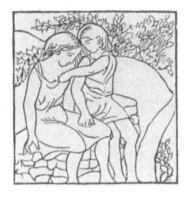

CHAPTER FIVE

The Joys of Sensual Touch

As predicted by many futurists, we are becoming more and more alienated from one another. The insanely fast pace of our lives combined with our habit of plunking ourselves down in front of the television or the computer to watch sitcoms or surf the Web for relaxation have caused many couples to become so distant they seldom talk to each other. And as a result we are desperately hungry for connection.

Nothing can provide that connection the way touch can. Nothing else can make up for what we are lacking—the sense of well-being, fulfillment, relaxation, and joy that can only come from human touch.

Touch can truly transform us from detached, unemotional, insecure beings into loving, connected, emotional ones. When you involve yourself in the touch exercises outlined in this chapter and throughout this book, your senses will be heightened, your sense of self-worth will be significantly increased, and your ability to respond and connect with others will improve tremendously.

☉ The Joys of Sensual Touch ☉

There are many ways other than sexual activity to have intimate contact, and many ways of expressing love for each other: holding hands, caressing and massaging, taking a bath or Jacuzzi together, or just cuddling. Yet most people focus exclusively on sex as a way of connecting. In fact, many of us have grown so accustomed to attempting to get all our needs for intimacy met through sex that we are unable to feel and express intimacy any other way.

Our skin is our body's largest organ, and our entire body, from the top of our heads to the soles of our feet, offers us a feast of potential sensual and erotic delights. Most of us, though, focus all our attention on our genitals when making love, even though there are other parts of the body that can be just as erotic and feel just as pleasurable when touched. Men in particular tend to focus all their attention on their penis and on ejaculation as opposed to intimacy and pleasure.

There is a continuum of sensual touch, progressing from less sexual to intensely sexual. This continuum begins with holding, hugging, and kissing and moves up to stroking, massage, and sexual pleasuring. By exploring a variety of ways of expressing intimacy, you and your partner will become less compulsive or goal oriented and more spontaneous and loving.

In addition, many people view foreplay strictly as a preliminary activity, a kind of appetizer with intercourse being the main course. But it doesn't have to be that way. Many couples reach satisfying sexual climax (including orgasm) through activities that are considered only foreplay, such as stimulating the genitals by hand, tongue, or mouth. These activities shouldn't be seen as any less "vital" than intercourse, and can be just as satisfying, or more so, for both partners.

The quantity and quality of our nonsexual touching experiences are intimately related to how satisfied we are with our sexual activities. "Why is this?" you might ask. "Just what does touching have to do with the quality of my sexual behavior?" The answer, according to Lonnie Barbach in her wonderful book *For Each Other,* is that for most people, sexual experiences are most fulfilling, and the chances of avoiding sexual problems is highest, when they have sex because they want sex—not something else. When you use sex in an attempt to satisfy nonsexual needs such as the need for comforting, reassurance, or physical contact, you run the risk of becoming disappointed. Sex that is motivated by other needs is often unsatisfying and can even lead to sexual problems, since our bodies usually respond to what we really want. If all you really want is a hug, your body may refuse to respond sexually to even the most erotic touches.

When you only share physical contact and affection in the context of sexual activity, sex takes on an exaggerated importance. It becomes weighed down with all the needs that aren't being met elsewhere. Ask yourself what you really want when you think you want sex. Is it closeness to someone you care about, a feeling of connectedness? Is it understanding or support? Is it reassurance that the person you care about cares about you in return? Or is it intercourse or orgasm?

Once you have some idea of what you want at any given time, ask your-self what the best way of getting it might be. Do you really just need a hug or to be held? Or do you need to connect with your partner by having an intimate conversation, perhaps including the request for some verbal reas-surance? How would giving or receiving a massage feel? If you begin to take the time to ask yourself these questions, you will find that you will also begin to get your sexual needs and desires fulfilled in lovemaking and sat-isfy needs for other kinds of contact and affection in more appropriate ways.

There will, of course, be times when sex is exactly what you want and need. But consider the following exercises for those times when sensual touch is a more appropriate way to satisfy your needs and desires.

⑥ Sensate Focus Exercises ⑩

The following exercises are called sensate focus exercises and originated with the work of the sex therapists Masters and Johnson. You already com-pleted one such exercise when you did the foot caress in the previous chap-ter. In my practice, these exercises have helped hundreds of couples suffer-ing from a variety of sexual and intimacy problems and are one of the most important parts of the book. You will find that I refer to them several times when I discuss the different phases of your relationship. By the end of the book I will have given you the complete sensate focus program. If you do nothing else I have suggested in this book, make sure you learn these exer-cises. Designed to help establish trust between couples and to help them find alternative ways of touching and sharing intimacy, they can change your life and your relationship.

The term *sensate focus* refers to the fact that during these exercises you are to focus your attention as closely as you can on your sensations, how it feels to touch or be touched. For example, whether you are the one giving the touch or receiving it, make sure that you always focus all your attention on the point where your body comes in contact with your partner's skin. If your mind wanders during the exercise, bring it back to the exact point of contact between your skin and your partner's.

This way of touching, called caressing, has been proven to remove the pressure to perform, to allow people to touch for their own pleasure, and to help people express tenderness, caring, and gentleness. The word *caress* comes from the Latin *carus,* which means "dear" or "precious." Caressing is a special way of touching that enables you to communicate to your lover just how dear he is to you, just how precious his body is to you. Using your hands as an extension of your heart, caressing will enable you to worship your loved one as only a lover can.

Caressing is different from massage or even what is commonly called "sensual massage," because instead of manipulating the underlying muscles of the body, you focus on the skin. Caressing is a slow, sensuous touch that is much lighter than massage and is done very, very slowly, using not just your fingertips but your entire hand and even your forearm. You caress your partner's skin with long sweeping strokes, using the flat of your fingers, palm, wrist, and forearm.

Another difference between caressing and massaging is that massage is intended solely for the pleasure or therapeutic benefit of the person receiving the massage, while caressing is done for the pleasure of the person giving the caress as well. You may have noticed in the past that you became easily tired while giving a massage and may even have become anxious because you were concerned about whether you were doing it right and pleasing the person to whom you were giving the massage. While the person receiving a caress certainly does enjoy it, the person giving the caress enjoys it just as much, and since you are not worried about how well you are performing, it will not feel like a task but a pleasure.

To understand exactly what I mean, try the following exercise.

Imagine that your right hand is the "giver" and that your left hand is the "receiver." Touch your left hand using only the fingertips of your right hand. Which of your hands feels the pleasure of the touch? Most people will say that their left hand, the "receiver," feels the pleasure. But what about your right hand—does it feel any pleasure? Most people say no, they don't feel any pleasure in using their fingertips.

Now try "giving" to the left hand using the flat of your right hand, wrist, and the flat of your fingers. Which hand feels the pleasure of the touch this time? Most people will say that both hands feel pleasure, both the "giver" and the "receiver." Indeed, it is hard to tell which hand is the "giver" and which is the "receiver" when you use the caress technique.

You and your partner may or may not choose to use a lotion or oil when caressing. Some people do not like the feel of lotion or oil on their skin, and some people, such as survivors of childhood sexual abuse, may have a negative association with lotion or oil, especially if their perpetrator used it. If you decide to use an oil or lotion, make sure it is one that both of you like. Pay particular attention to the fragrance and make certain it does not elicit negative memories for either one of you. (See chapter 4 for more information on massage oils.)

Always do the exercises in a private, quiet environment. Take the phone off the hook, send the children to a baby-sitter, or wait until the kids are in bed at night. Some people prefer to have some easy-listening music, but it is really best to do these exercises in silence. It is far too easy to become distracted by music, and your intention here is to focus on touch only.

Exercise | **When You Are the Active Partner**

Always maintain contact with your partner as you are giving the caress to avoid startling her with a sudden touch when you switch hands. If you use lotion or oil, warm it in your hand before you apply it, and maintain contact with your partner's body when you reapply the lotion.

You can use long, sweeping strokes using your forearm, wrist, palm of your hand, and flat of your fingers, or you can alternate with shorter strokes, using only the flat of your fingers. Make sure that you do not use your fingertips, however, because they can tickle your partner.

Make sure that you are going very, very slowly, the slower the better. If you think you are moving your hand slowly enough, cut your speed in half and see how this affects your ability to focus on the touch. Do not worry about whether your partner is enjoying the caress. It will be his or her responsibility to let you know if you are doing something uncomfortable. Since sensate focus exercises are intended to promote relaxation, both you and your partner will feel more relaxed if the exercises are done very slowly, with both of you closing your eyes.

While it is normal to become distracted now and then, if you find your mind wandering, try bringing it back to the place where your skin makes contact with your partner's skin.

Do not speak or ask for feedback during the exercise. Assume that the caress feels good or at least neutral.

Exercise | **When You Are the Passive Partner**

Close your eyes and try to relax any muscles that feel tense. Keep your attention on the place where your partner is touching your skin. Mentally follow your partner's hand as it caresses your body. Do not give your partner any feedback unless something feels painful or uncomfortable. Do not moan or groan or wiggle around, because this can be a subtle way of manipulating the active partner into continuing to touch a particular spot. Remaining completely passive will allow your body to experience pleasure more fully. If you become tense, try taking some deep breaths to relax yourself and focus only on the touch.

Because it may be hard to remember all these instructions, here is a summary of things to keep in mind while doing the sensate focusing exercises:

1. Agree on the limits of the exercise beforehand and do not go beyond those limits.

2. Always focus on the point of contact where your skin touches your partner's skin.

3. When you are active, do the exercise for your own pleasure and do not worry whether your partner is enjoying it. Use a slow, light caressing technique.

4. Stay passive when in the passive role—do not give feedback.

5. Focus on sensual pleasure rather than on sexual arousal.

6. If anxiety—yours or your partner's—does not quickly decrease after the first few minutes of an exercise, stop the exercise immediately.

7. Don't work at it. Relax.

8. Provide honest feedback after the exercise.

E x e r c i s e | **Self-Caressing**

In preparation for the sensate focus exercises you will do later with your partner, begin practicing sensual caressing on yourself. This will help you discover how you like to be touched, which will be invaluable when you begin to communicate your desires to your partner. Also, the more you learn about your own body responses, the more you will increase your ability to become aroused. Finally, by becoming increasingly receptive to your own body you will become more loving toward your partner's body.

It is normal to feel a little self-conscious caressing yourself, especially when you move to your genitals, but with practice you will soon become comfortable with it.

❖ *Begin by choosing a small area of the body, such as an arm, a thigh, or your chest for your first self-caress. Warm some oil in the palm of your hand and slowly begin to caress yourself. Use a slow, light touch. Remember that the emphasis is sensual rather than sexual. Focus all your attention on the point of contact between your hand and your body. If your mind starts to wander, bring it back to noticing how your skin feels. Notice the temperature and texture of your skin. Add more oil if your skin feels dry. If you still have trouble concentrating, slow down your touch.*

❖ *Continue caressing yourself in this way for at least ten minutes, paying particular attention to how it feels when you use the flats of your fingers, your palms, your wrists, and your forearms. Which of these touches do you prefer? Can you imagine how good it would feel to your partner to be touched in this way?*

❖ *Move on to exploring the rest of your body. Be creative, caressing your knees, ears, face. Which parts of your body feel the best when caressed?*

Exercise | **Genital Self-Caressing**

Now you will move on to a genital caress. This will be very different from masturbation in that the goal is not to turn yourself on or to have an orgasm but to discover what kind of touch you prefer on your genitals.

❖ *Take all your clothes off and lie down in a comfortable position. Put some oil or other lubricant on your hand and begin to slowly touch your inner thighs. If any part of your body is tense, make a conscious effort to relax. Concentrate all your attention on the point of contact between your hand and your body and move very slowly, just as you did in the previous exercise.*

❖ *Women, begin to touch your labia and your clitoris. Try different types of touches, such as the kind your partner usually uses to touch you and the kind you usually use to touch yourself. Now try a completely different type of touch.*

   Do not spend most of the time on your clitoris but experiment with all areas of your genitals. Pay attention to the different textures and temperatures as you touch various areas. Which is the most sensitive? Which is most arousing?

   Keep your breathing even and relax your muscles. If you become sexually aroused, that's fine, but it is not the goal. Continue for at least fifteen minutes. If you have an orgasm, fine, but don't try to make it happen.

❖ *Men, follow the instructions for women, except obviously you will be caressing your penis and scrotum. Remember that this is different from masturbating, since the goal is to learn what type of touch you prefer. If your mind begins to wander at any given point, especially if you begin to fantasize, slow the movement and bring your focus to the exact point of contact between your fingers and your genitals. Notice the different textures and temperatures of the skin. Experiment with different types of touch. Keep your muscles relaxed and breathe evenly. If you begin to approach orgasm, do nothing to make it happen or push it away, but just allow it to happen. Continue this exercise for at least fifteen minutes.*

Practice these self-caressing exercises a few more times before you begin doing the exercises with your partner. They will teach you how to do the caress technique, how to pay attention to the kind of touch you prefer, how to breathe into arousal, and how to relax muscles, all important aspects of Sensual Sex.

⑥ The Back and Front Caress ⑥

The following exercises should bring you much closer together than you have ever been before and add to your repertoire of sensual ways of sharing. In addition, they will help to build trust and provide each person with a feeling of being loved.

These exercises also include a time set aside for verbal feedback. Practicing giving such feedback can help tremendously in your efforts to communicate your sexual needs.

Exercise | **The Back Caress**

Preparation: You will need massage oil, a large beach towel, a bath towel, and some paper towels. As always, you will need a quiet room where you will not be disturbed, with a bed or some other comfortable surface that offers plenty of room for both of you to stretch out on.

The back caress includes the entire back of the body from the neck to the feet. It is normally done in the nude, but for those who are uncomfortable being completely nude in front of your partner, I recommend you both wear shorts, bathing suits, or underwear. Women may feel comfortable in a halter top or a bra.

The passive partner should lie comfortably, face down, with a towel underneath. He may keep his arms at his sides or underneath his head, whichever is most comfortable. The active person should lie or sit next to the passive partner without leaning on him.

The active person begins to caress the passive person's back with one hand, beginning at the neck. Slowly run your palm or your fingers over the shoulder blades and then down the spine.

Remember, this is not a massage. The object is to use your hand to find areas that feel particularly good to you.

Continue touching your partner, moving slowly down the back to the buttocks and legs. Remember to stroke your partner slowly, and try to keep your eyes closed when at all possible to enhance your pleasure and to maximize your ability to focus on physical sensations. If you have difficulty focusing, slow down and bring your mind back to the exact point of contact between your skin and your partner's skin.

Pay attention to how the various parts of your partner's body feel when you caress them with your palm, wrist, and forearm instead of just your fingertips. When you find that a particular part of the body feels especially good to you, savor the touch and linger there awhile. Pay attention to the various textures and temperatures in different parts of the body.

There should be no sexual touching during this exercise. Do not reach between your partner's legs and attempt to caress the genitals. Do not try to place your hands between her buttocks. Your partner must be able to feel completely safe knowing that you are not going to go beyond the limits of the exercise.

If you notice that your partner is tensing up, remind her to breathe and relax and continue with the caress.

Each person should spend approximately twenty to thirty minutes doing the back caress. Complete the caress by making long, smooth strokes starting at your partner's shoulders and moving all the way down to her feet. You may want to indicate that you have finished by firmly placing your hands on the bottom of her feet.

When you are the passive partner, make yourself comfortable, breathe deeply, and relax your muscles. Keep your mind on the exact point of contact where your partner is touching you. Try not to move; just passively soak up the sensations. The only time you need to communicate with your partner is if she does something that hurts you or makes you uncomfortable.

If you become sexually aroused either as the giver or the receiver during the back caress, fine. Just enjoy the arousal and bring your mind back to the point of contact.

Feedback: When You Are the Active Partner

After you have completed the back caress, lie or sit down by your partner and give her plenty of time to take in the deep sensual pleasure and relaxation that she experienced. Take this time to recall your own reactions. How are you feeling now that the exercise is complete? Do you feel tired or relaxed and rejuvenated? How do you feel toward your partner? Do you feel more loving? More intimate? Do you feel sexually aroused?

Once your partner has begun to stir, ask her to begin giving you feedback about her experience. Listen carefully, but do not interrupt. Allow her to express all her feelings before sharing your own.

When your partner gets to the part where she is giving you feedback about what she liked the most, listen extra carefully and make a mental note for future reference. Finally, when she gives you feedback about what made her uncomfortable, try not to get defensive. Don't try to explain yourself or make excuses; just listen so that in the future you will not repeat the same action.

Feedback: When You Are the Passive Partner

After your partner has completed the back caress, lie quietly, taking in all the wonderful feelings you've experienced. Don't rush to get up; allow yourself to relax and fully connect with your body and emotions.

When you are ready, begin to move your body ever so slowly. Carefully and gently roll over so that you are facing your partner. Cover yourself if you are cold or self-conscious and sit up if you feel like it.

Share with your partner what the experience was like for you, including what part of your body you enjoyed having touched the most (your shoulders? the top part of your back? your buttocks? your legs?) and what kind of stroke you liked the best (long, smooth strokes? firm, deep strokes? soft, gentle strokes?). Now tell your partner how you felt emotionally about receiving this caress from him. Share any deep feelings that were evoked, such as love, pain, or guilt. For example, did you feel more loved by your partner than you have felt in a long time, did you have a difficult time accepting this caress, did you begin to feel like you didn't deserve it?

Finally, gently but firmly tell your partner about anything that made you uncomfortable, anything that you would prefer he not do the next time. For example, did he spent a lot more time on your buttocks than on any other part of the body and did you feel this as subtle sexual pressure? Did he tend to lean on your body too much, making you uncomfortable? Or did you feel that he began to tire or get bored and was rushing to get the exercise over with? (Make sure you check this out with your partner, since we can sometimes misinterpret others' actions.)

Exercise | **Front Caress**

The front caress includes the entire front of the body, from the neck to the feet. Follow the same instructions for preparation, caressing, and feedback as given for the back caress above.

Special consideration needs to be given to the fact that the woman's breasts and both partner's genitals are exposed during this exercise. This can make some people feel especially self-conscious. Although this exercise is normally done in the nude, if either one of you is too uncomfortable you may wear underwear, bathing suits, or shorts, or place a towel over whatever area makes you feel vulnerable.

Since the purpose of this exercise is not to stimulate your partner sexually, you should treat the genitals and nipples as you would any other part of the body, and not give them special attention. A man should caress the woman's breasts as he would any other part of her body, not ignoring the nipples but not touching them differently from how he touches the rest of the body. The same holds true for women with regard to the penis. Do not avoid the penis entirely but do not pick it up and begin manipulating it with your hands and fingers. Try using your palm, wrist, and forearm to briefly make long, sweeping motions across it.

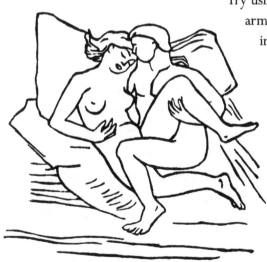

Many men will get erections before and during the time their penis is being caressed, and women's nipples will undoubtedly become aroused. This is normal and is not a signal for you to begin stimulating them still further. It is also normal for a man to remain so relaxed that he doesn't get an erection, or for his erection to come and go throughout the exercise. Try to make no assumptions about the significance of the state of a man's penis or a woman's nipples whatsoever.

Once again, as you did with the back caress, complete the caress by making long, smooth strokes, starting at your partner's shoulders and moving all the way down to her feet. Lie together for a few minutes taking in the experience before beginning feedback.

E x e r c i s e | **The Sexual Caress**

The sexual caress flows from the body caress and should be done following a full-body caress, at least in the beginning, when you are learning the technique. Later on, you can do it as a prelude to lovemaking.

When the male is the active partner:

❖ *Have your partner lie on her stomach with her thighs spread apart.*

❖ *Begin by caressing the insides of her thighs, starting at her knees. Using your forearms, wrists, and palms make a slow, sensuous movement up the inside of her thighs, up and over her buttock to the small of her back.*

❖ *Now reverse your movements but this time concentrate on the outside of her body. Begin at the small of the back, moving down the outside of her buttocks to the outside of her thighs.*

❖ *Repeat the entire cycle several times until the movement feels like one long, continuous, flowing stroke—up the inside of her thighs, over her buttocks to the small of her back, then down the outside of her buttocks and the outside of her thighs to her knees.*

❖ *Have your partner turn over, and follow the same procedure on the front of her body with emphasis again on the inside of her thighs, up over her genitals, over her stomach to her chest. Apply a particularly light touch to her nipples, areola, and breast tissues, emphasizing a greater sensual and sexual feeling than was present during the body caress but do not linger. Continue to use the flat of your fingers, your* palms, wrist, and forearm, as opposed to your fingertips. Now once again reverse your movements as you caress down the outside of her body to her thighs. Once again, repeat the entire cycle several times— up the inside of her thighs, over her pubic mound, up the middle of her stomach, to the middle of her chest, then down the outside of her chest and stomach all the way back again to the outside of her thighs.

❖ The last phase of the sexual caress is for you to lubricate your index finger and use it to massage your lover's genitals. Gently touch the outer lips, then the inner lips, and finally the clitoris. Notice the different textures of the skin and the various temperatures of different parts of the genitals. Touch for your own pleasure, as well as your partner's. Spend at least five minutes gently stimulating these areas before inserting your finger very slowly into the vagina. Do not begin thrusting but instead gently caress the inside of her vagina with your finger. The purpose of the exercise is to bring pleasure to you and your partner. If orgasm occurs, fine, but don't push for it.

When the female is the active partner:

❖ Have your partner lie on his stomach with his legs spread apart.

❖ Follow the directions above except that when you have your partner turn over on his back after you have completed caressing the front of his body, you will focus your attention on caressing his penis and scrotum. After warming some oil in your hand, slowly begin to lightly pleasure your partner's scrotum. Your touch should be light, and it is okay to use the tips of your fingers. Experiment with different touches, and pay attention to the different textures and temperatures. Now slowly begin to caress the shaft and then the head of his penis. Try not to use your fingertips, but stimulate your partner using the flat of your fingers, your palms, wrists, and even your forearm. Get into the experience for your own enjoyment as well as for your partner's. Your purpose is not to bring your partner to orgasm but if it occurs, fine. If your partner ejaculates before you have completed the exercise, simply wipe him off gently and continue.

Practicing sensual caressing will enable you to experience a deep connection with your partner, a connection far deeper than you have ever experienced before. By learning how to touch in a truly sensuous way you will learn to give each other pleasure beyond your wildest dreams. By learning all you can about your partner's body, every curve and every angle, you will be able to play your partner's body like an instrument, creating music together that touches your souls. And by learning how to receive touch, by learning how to truly take in the pleasure, you will be able to experience a level of vulnerability and openness that you may have previously believed impossible.

⑤ Sensuality for One ⑨

At this point some of you may still be experiencing resistance from your partner and may have been unable to do the sensate focus exercises together. Don't despair. You don't have to miss out on romance, sensuality, and sexual excitement just because your partner is not willing to participate at this time. You can have the excitement and fulfillment of a full sex life if you are willing to do the following: learn to look within for the source of your orgasmic joy, learn to love yourself as you are, including loving your body just as it is. And last but not least, treat yourself as you would a lover.

A woman I only knew briefly told me how she had decided to "take herself on as a lover" as a way of maintaining her sex life even though she was single. What she meant by this was that she actively behaved as if she were her own lover, treating herself in the way she would like a lover to treat her—setting the stage with satin sheets, candlelight, and music that she found very erotic.

Once a week, preferably when you are very relaxed and have plenty of time, make a date with yourself for a sexual encounter, just as you would if you had a date. You might choose a night when your husband works late and the kids aren't at home. Or you may want to wait until everyone is in bed. Your date might begin with a sensuous candlelit dinner with soft

music. Choose your food carefully, making elegant choices of either sensuous, erotic food (sushi, artichokes) or light and healthy food (salad, fish,
vegetables). Eat slowly, savoring each bite, enjoying the texture and aroma
of the food as much as you enjoy the taste.

Set the stage for your sexual encounter by making the room as erotic as
possible. If you are a romantic, try candlelight, flowers, and scented sheets.
If you are more boisterous, you might choose rock and roll or heavy metal
music, neon lights, and black satin sheets. Taking a long, sensuous bath is
another way of relaxing and preparing for your sexual encounter, while
some prefer a sensuous shower. Try the self-caressing exercises described
in this chapter before you begin masturbating, or skip masturbation if you
aren't in the mood and focus instead on feeding your senses.

Hopefully, it won't be long before your partner responds to your
overtures for sensuous connecting. In the meantime, don't deprive yourself
of a sensuous life. You deserve to treat yourself as sensuously, as lavishly
as you would treat a romantic partner. You deserve to make your house,
and your bedroom especially, as sensuous and erotic as you would if
you had company. And you deserve to use the finest massage and essential
oils to help make your self-touching experience one that is nurturing,
stimulating, and fulfilling.

Sacred sex, which is the experience of ecstasy,

is the real sexual revolution.

— GEORG FEUERSTEIN

The soul should always stand ajar,

ready to welcome the ecstatic experience.

— EMILY DICKINSON

Through sex we enter the timeless,

boundary-less moment. We partake

of the one experience above all

others in life which allows us

the bliss of true union.

— DAPHNE ROSE KINGMA

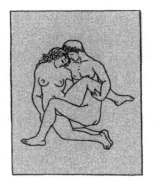

CHAPTER SIX

Deeper Love

We all desire to love and be loved in a deep, meaningful way, to know the kind of love that touches our very souls. Unfortunately, many of us are too cut off from our emotions to be able to experience such a love. We become frightened of our deeper feelings and retreat into the safety of superficiality. Or we don't take the time to develop deeper love but instead look around for a new thrill, a new love.

In many relationships sex is so mechanical and routine that there is no feeling, no real soul. Sadly, many still view the sex act simply as a biological chore—and not a very pleasant one. For others, sex, when it occurs (twice a week on the average, according to research) is a brief encounter that leaves both partners feeling unfulfilled and unloved. Even their orgasmic release feels like a letdown; because although two people may be having sex, they may not be having sex together. And while their bodies may be connecting, there is no emotional and spiritual exchange.

Many women have become experts at faking orgasms to deal with pressure from lovers, who insist that they climax every time. Some couples even become obsessed with climaxing at the same time, and some women have become such firm believers in multiple orgasms that they insist that their partner gratify their desire by becoming a thrusting machine. All these attitudes have created tremendous performance anxiety in both sexes, leading to sexual dysfunction, an inability to have orgasms, and sometimes sexual burnout—the feeling that sex is a frustrating experience and a source of conflict and emotional pain, something to be avoided at all costs.

To get away from routine sex, some men and women seek sexual and emotional fulfillment with partners outside their relationship. Usually this only leads to further disappointment, because sex cannot be isolated from the rest of our lives. Sex outside one's established relationship is seldom fulfilling and may in fact add to one's overall stress. There are also some who attempt to overcome their boredom by exploring alternative sex (for example, bondage, sadomasochism, group sex). Few find what they are really looking for—the fulfillment that can only come from intimate lovemaking.

More and more people are discovering that fulfillment cannot be found in the sex act alone, however frequent, varied, or momentarily relieving it may be. Many, especially women, are beginning to express their desire for greater intimacy in their sexual relationships. Routine sex depersonalizes both partners. For lovemaking to be fulfilling, all of you must be involved, not just your genitals. Sex with a partner with whom you share no other connection can often be empty and meaningless. Sensual Sex, however, helps bring couples together in ways that are both exciting and meaningful, helping them to reach deeper levels of intimacy.

Being intimate means being open and vulnerable, to each other and to your own feelings. To be sexually vulnerable you must be willing to relinquish control—both mentally and physically. You must be able to trust your partner enough to go with what gives you pleasure without hesitation.

Also, to obtain greater intimacy and deeper love, you and your partner will need to go deeper into yourselves—deeper into your emotions, deeper into your bodily sensations. Without deep feeling, without participation of the heart, all the modern and ancient sex techniques combined will not lead to complete satisfaction and connection.

In this chapter you will learn ways to become more vulnerable, to deepen your emotional intimacy and your love. We will begin by discussing the importance of deep breathing and techniques such as Deep Breathing and Synchronized Breathing. Then you will be encouraged to deepen your relationship by opening up to what is commonly called "sacred sex," or the achievement of a spiritual connection with your partner during sex. I will include a brief discussion of the philosophy of tantric sex and some of its techniques. You will learn in this chapter that sex is never boring when you make love to each other's souls.

Throughout this chapter you will learn a variety of skills, many of which you will no doubt find useful. At the same time, I would like to stress that the most valuable and authentic lovemaking skill is allowing yourself to feel, really feel, both physically and emotionally.

⑤ Deep Breathing ⑤

When we were babies we all breathed in an instinctive way that was nat-ural and complete. To see this natural way of breathing in action, watch a healthy baby. You will notice that the baby breathes from both his chest and belly.

As we grow older and our bodies become more rigid (from fear, trauma, and defensiveness), we tend to alter this natural way of breathing. Most of us begin to breathe only from our chests, though some breathe only from their bellies. We also begin to breathe shallowly instead of deeply. This type of breathing often results from muscular tensions that build up over years. Many of us are taught as children to stand up straight and to push our chest out and pull our belly in, and this rigid posture tight-ens our breathing muscles.

In addition, we may have also unconsciously restricted our breathing as a way of suppressing painful emotions, using shallow breathing as an anes-thetic. Although this is very effective when handling a crisis, when shallow breathing becomes habitual, we often end up cutting off our ability to feel all our emotions, the "positive" ones as well as the "negative." For example, both women and men tend to hold their breath during sex. This is usually a sign of tension, and interferes with the ability to fully experience sensual and sexual pleasure.

The techniques of complete or deep breathing given below can help us to breathe deeply and to regain the balance of breathing from both our chests and our bellies.

Complete Breath

A complete breath consists of four stages:
1. inhalation
2. retention
3. exhalation
4. pause

The art of working with these stages is highly developed in the Taoist and hatha yoga schools, and yet all this practice begins with learning complete breath. While this type of breathing may at first seem strange, it will quickly begin to feel much more natural than your old way of breathing.

* *Sit erect but comfortable, with your hands on your hips or in your lap.*

* *Close your eyes.*

* *Breathe through your nose.*

* *Relax.*

* *Now consciously draw your breath deeply into the back of your throat and allow it to flow down against your spine.*

* *Allow your breath to go all the way down until it can't go any further and naturally flows upward into your lower belly and navel.*

* *When your belly is comfortably full, allow the air to rise and to expand your ribs.*

* *Let your chest rise. If your shoulders rise a little, that's okay.*

* *Just as you filled yourself from bottom to top, now empty yourself from top to bottom, from chest to belly.*

* *Compress the chest firmly, using your hand at first. Let your shoulders down.*

* *Exhale very slowly and gently.*

* *Allow your belly to deflate automatically.*

* *You have just completed one full breath.*

Simple Deep Breathing

Even though Complete Breath is the ideal way to breathe, it can be difficult to learn. If you find the directions too complicated or are unwilling to put that much effort into learning it, try this alternative.

❖ *Lie comfortably on your back with your clothing loosened.*

❖ *Place your hand on your abdomen.*

❖ *Take a deep breath. To breathe freely, your belly should be relaxed and your shoulders down. In addition, your diaphragm, the dome-shaped sheet of muscle that separates the lungs from the abdominal organs, needs to be flexible.*

❖ *Exhale, blowing all the air in your lungs out through your mouth.*

❖ *Notice whether your stomach goes up or down. Typically, when we breathe most of us do the opposite of what is really natural—our stomach goes in when we inhale and out when we exhale. For natural, deep breathing, the stomach should extend when we inhale and contract when we exhale. Try to breathe in this way a few times, using your hand as an indicator.*

❖ *Now take several breaths, making sure your stomach presses up against your hand when you inhale and sinks away from your hand as you exhale. Slowly breathe in through your mouth, and then immediately, but slowly, exhale. Pause several seconds between exhaling and inhaling. Do not pause between an inhalation and an exhalation. The inhale/exhale movement should be one continuous process. Practice breathing like this for a few minutes.*

The most important things to remember are to breathe slowly, deeply, and evenly. By breathing in this way you will allow sexual energy to flow throughout your body and you will increase your concentration, thus allowing yourself to be more present during lovemaking.

Synchronized Deep Breathing

Couples often talk about their desire to become one, to flow together and to get in rhythm with each other. There is no better way to achieve this than by practicing synchronized breathing, which can increase your feelings of connection and harmony with your partner.

Breathing together is also a beautiful way to communicate nonverbally. Synchronized deep breathing at any stage of lovemaking will intensify both your feelings and your energy level. And deep breathing together as you are approaching orgasm can help create an incredibly exciting experience.

Partners can breathe together in two ways. You can breathe in and out as one, or you can alternate like two pistons, with one breathing in as the other breathes out. The first is breathing simultaneously, the second is breathing in tandem.

Try this technique.

❖ *Sit facing each other. Make eye contact and begin to breathe together, inhaling and exhaling at the same time. Decide who will be the leader and who will be the follower. The leader will begin breathing very slowly and deeply, and the follower will emulate her breathing pattern until you are breathing in sync with one another. Notice how it feels to breathe deeply, how relaxed it makes you feel, and how it feels to breathe together in this way.*

❖ *Now the leader should speed up her breathing and the follower will match her breath. Notice how much more excited you tend to feel when you breathe more rapidly and how it feels to breathe together.*

Generally speaking, fast breathing is associated with feeling excited and slow breathing is associated with feeling calm. This exercise also shows you how one partner's breathing can have a particular effect on his partner and how two people can breathe together to achieve a desired state of arousal or relaxation.

Exercise | **Spoon Breathing**

The purpose of this exercise is to help you relax, but it is also an ideal way for lovers to connect, to pay attention to each other's responses, and to get in sync. It is an excellent technique to use before doing any of the caressing exercises offered in the book, before lovemaking, or as a way to reconnect after an argument or estrangement.

Lie together on a comfortable bed or couch with one person's back snuggled up against the other person's front, bending your legs so that you fit together like two spoons. Lie very still without talking for a few minutes. Then the person in back places her hand on the stomach of the one in front. This is a signal that she is now ready to follow the breathing of her partner. The person in front begins to breathe deeply, and the person in the back adjusts her breathing to match his.

Our ability to experience the richness and intensity of our emotions is closely related to the depth of our breathing. By continuing to practice deep breathing, you will continue to free the flow of energy in your body, which in turn will increase your capacity for pleasure and your ability to express love.

⑤ Erotic Awakening ⑤

In addition to the breathing exercises above, the following Erotic Awakening techniques can also deepen your passion and increase your level of intimacy.

Erotic Awakening encourages you to take hours worshiping and adoring your lover's body. It also requires you to go completely beyond all your conventional notions about foreplay and arousal. In these exercises you will need to act and feel as if giving the awakening touch is the climax, that genital union does not exist. Paradoxically, when genital intercourse eventually takes place, you will experience more fulfillment than you ever imagined possible.

As you arouse your partner, you will awaken her as though from a deep sleep of boredom into vivid expanded vibrating aliveness. You will penetrate self-protective layers with your life-giving touch, bringing your partner into the present and into vitality.

Exercise | **Awakening Touch**

Ask your lover to lie on a bed or massage table, naked and face down. Touch her very lightly all over her body, communicating your love through your hands. You can use your fingertips for this touch, but also remember to use the flat of your fingers and the palm of your hand. Do not press down on your lover's skin but instead allow your hand to hover above it, just barely touching. Your touch should be so light that she can barely feel it. Move extremely slowly, so slowly that it will take at least a half-hour to complete the Awakening Touch on each side of the body. Make sure that you are breathing deeply throughout the exercise, and that you are touching with love in your heart. Focus on the energy coming from your hands and concentrate on making it move into your lover's body.

Once you have completed touching her entire body, front and back, have your lover turn over once again so she is face down. Position yourself at your lover's head and, without touching her, breathe on her as you move down her body. Begin by breathing on her neck and shoulders, then her back, buttocks, and legs.

Now ask your lover to turn over, so she is face up. Breathe on her face, in her ears, on her neck. Imagine that your breath is infusing your lover with energy. Move down to her shoulders, arms, and chest. Take a few moments to breathe your love into her heart area. Summon up your deepest feelings of love as you breathe onto her stomach, her hips, her pelvic area. Let your hot breath heat up her genitals and inner thighs. Move all the way down her legs to her feet, finishing your breath caress by breathing on the soles of her feet.

After a pause, switch roles so that you are now the passive partner. As your lover lightly touches you all over your body, feel the love that is being communicated and take it into your heart. Breathe deeply and focus on feeling the energy coming from your partner's hands into your body. Take in the energy and love as your partner breathes them into your body.

After you have each had a turn being the active and passive partner, face each other and look deeply into each other's eyes.

Continue touching in the same loving, sensuous way for at least fifteen more minutes.

Spreading

Spreading is a technique developed to help spread feelings of arousal and sexual energy from the genitals to the rest of the body. If we focus all our attention on the genitals when making love, this not only puts a lot of pressure on ourselves and our partner to reach orgasm but also deprives us of being able to feel the sexual arousal all over our body. Spreading helps us to hold the charge of sexual energy, which in turn enhances our lovemaking. Many also experience this total, yet relaxed, arousal as an ecstatic encounter.

While the "passive" partner in all the exercises is never really passive, since he or she is focusing on breathing, relaxing, and noticing sensations, in Spreading, the physically passive partner will be particularly active internally as he feels and directs the sexual energy from his genitals to other parts of his body.

❖ *As the passive partner you will lie face up on the bed, genitals exposed. To ensure maximum relaxation, keep your palms up, with your arms at about a forty-five-degree angle to your torso and your feet slightly apart. Relax your jaw so that your teeth are slightly separated.*

❖ *As the active partner, stand or kneel by the side of the bed and begin slowly caressing your partner's body all over, using long strokes. Use an oil if you wish. Although you will be using the gentle caressing strokes you have already learned in previous chapters, at the end of each long stroke gradually decrease the pressure even more until your hand is actually an inch or so above your partner's body. Spend at least a full ten minutes doing this.*

❖ *Begin to stimulate your partner's genitals until he is clearly aroused. Now "spread" the arousal to the rest of his body by using long, brushing strokes to "sweep" the energy away from the genitals, down the legs, and toward the feet. At the end of each stroke gradually lessen the pressure of your touch, ending with leaving your partner's body briefly but completely.*

❖ *Return to the genitals and once again gently caress to arousal. Now repeat the spreading stroke, moving away from the genitals but this time toward the head.*

❖ *Do this three or four times in each direction. Use long, smooth, light strokes, always tapering off to almost no pressure and then to hovering about an inch over the body with no contact.*

❖ *Repeat the entire cycle again, starting with the genitals and spreading first to the feet and then toward the head. Then switch roles.*

❖ *The passive person should remember to breathe deeply and slowly throughout the Spreading exercise. Focus on feeling and spreading the sexual energy throughout your body.*

There are variations to this spreading technique, such as incorporating it into your lovemaking as a type of foreplay. Touch, kiss, and lick to achieve arousal, then begin spreading the energy.

Many couples prefer a form of informal spreading such as stimulating your partner's genitals and then reaching out to touch another part of the body. You will practice a form of this when you do the genital caress later on.

Spreading arousal leads, over time, to an awakening of the body's primal energy and is an effective way to enhance your ability to receive, enjoy, and sustain great amounts of ecstatic energy. By surrendering to the subtle, vibratory sensations as they occur, your usual sense of being confined to the body melts away. At whatever level you wish to approach it, Spreading can help bring you and your partner closer together emotionally.

⑤ Deeper Connections ⑤

The following suggestions and exercises will help you to connect deeply with your partner. Some of them will take some getting used to, while others will automatically feel natural. All are important tools to add to your daily sexual repertoire, tools that will help you along your journey to more passionate, intimate sharing.

Maintaining Eye Contact

Another way to deepen your relationship is to look into each other's eyes more often. This includes making eye contact while you are talking or when you have just a few minutes to connect on a busy day. Taking a few moments to silently sit together and look into each other's eyes before engaging in lovemaking will set the tone for deeper and more open sharing.

When you want to experience the deepest connection possible, maintain eye contact during lovemaking. When you close your eyes during sex you have a primarily individual experience. You are also more likely to fantasize when your eyes are closed. Those who risk looking into each other's eyes during sex remain more in the moment and experience a powerful connection with their partner.

It can be frightening to be so vulnerable, to let another person in so much, but it is worth the risk. Share your fears with your partner about being so open and ease into it a little at a time until it becomes more comfortable.

Maintaining eye contact while you orgasm can be especially frightening, but resist the impulse to close your eyes or turn away. Instead, allow your partner to really see you in those moments of complete vulnerability and surrender. This will encourage both of you to continue to open up in other ways.

Later on in this chapter we will talk about sacred sex and the role that maintaining eye contact can have in achieving a deeper, more spiritual connection with your partner.

Creating a Sensual Ritual

As I discussed at the beginning of this book, many of us have been desensi-
tized by our fast-paced lives, living with both real violence and the violence
we see on television every night. And in our modern, highly mechanized,
computer-driven, ecologically destructive world we have also begun to
lose touch with our souls.

One way to regain our feelings and recapture our souls is through the
time-honored strategy known as *ritual*. Ritual helps us to cut through emotional straitjackets and get to our core. To step out of a routine of disconnected sex, conduct a ritual before beginning any sexual activity. While routine conjures up mindless repetition, ritual signifies specialness and conscious intent. Sexual ritual helps us to meet each other heart to heart, soul
to soul.

Take the time to acknowledge and honor your partner before coming
together sexually. Your ritual may be as simple as lighting a candle and looking into each other's eyes, or it could be more elaborate, such as playing a
particular song, lighting incense, reciting poetry, reading quotations, reading passages from the Bible, or giving each other a sensual caress. Prepare
a ritual that is meaningful to you both, including elements from your reli-
gion, culture, marriage vows, or your history together. The key is to create
an atmosphere that will evoke a blend of wonder, reverence for life, and
playfulness.

By honoring your partner when you come together sexually, you create an emotional space for intimacy. Although it is important to create a ritual that has particular meaning to you as a couple, the following ideas may spark your creativity.

❖ *Prepare a sensual environment, keeping romance foremost in your mind. Include flowers, prepare a table with fruit, wine, and other succulent delicacies. Make sure there are no interruptions. Wear exotic yet comfortable clothing such as caftans, kimonos, or elegant robes.*

❖ *Bathe or shower separately, and then anoint each other with oil. Play no music except at the very beginning of the ritual.*

❖ *Sit facing each other with your eyes closed at first. Spend five minutes in silence, individually contemplating the depth of the love you have for each other or your highest wish for your relationship. Consciously focus on opening your heart to your lover.*

❖ *After about five minutes, open your eyes and maintain eye contact as you synchronize your breathing. Begin by breathing simultaneously and then switch to breathing in tandem.*

❖ *Open your eyes and express your deepest love and respect for each other with a simple statement such as "I love you and want only the best for you" or "You complete me" or "I honor the spirit of God within you."*

❖ *Take turns reading a short prayer or a selection of poetry, or play a musical selection, with the intent of expressing your love and opening your hearts to each other.*

Creating a sensual ritual can deepen your relationship and make your lovemaking more meaningful. It can also put new life into a relationship. Don't be afraid to experiment and to add elements to your ritual from time to time. Be creative and, above all, be light and easy. While it is good to take preparing for the ritual seriously, once you have started be playful and have fun.

Later on in this chapter we will discuss further suggestions for rituals, including those that precede tantric sex.

Slow Sex

Slow Sex is both an exercise and a way to make love. As an exercise, one of its greatest benefits is that it tends to increase your sensory awareness. You may notice many new things about your partner—the softness of her belly, the slight down on her cheeks, the muscles on the side of his neck, the freckles on his lips.

Slow Sex is exactly what its name implies. As you make love, move as slowly as possible. By barely moving and by allowing yourself to become completely motionless at times, you allow space for deeper intimacy to grow. You will also discover that your next impulse to move will be far more spontaneous and will originate from deep within you, rather than from trying to create a desired result or moving in the way you think would please your partner. As your instincts take over, you will discover a greater depth in your lovemaking, perhaps greater than you had ever imagined, because you will be moving from a deeper part of yourself.

This way of lovemaking can be quite difficult at first. Therefore, it is a good idea to agree ahead of time to make love in slow motion for a specific time. Most people begin with only five minutes. As you become more accustomed to it you will be able to continue for twenty to forty minutes, the ideal interval.

You can use Slow Sex as a prelude to your regular lovemaking, to sensitize you or as a way of slowing things down—as the following poem suggests.

MAKE YOUR LOVE LONG

Luxuriate in your lover's body,
Don't rush as if completing some task—
    Making a bed or diapering a baby.
Your lover's body is your temple in which to worship your love,
Your canvas on which to create your bliss.
Use long, slow strokes to create the colors of your love,
    Your lust.

Round out the sharp edges of your beloved's life,
Revitalize the tired muscles, the hungry skin.
Breathe life back into the hollows of your love's sacred heart,
Your lover's pulsating center of joy.

Your beloved's body is a precious gift,
Smell the sweetness of skin made all the sweeter by your love,
Get lost in tangled hair,
Entwine your arms and legs like ripened vines,
Taste the salt of sweat and tears, the sap of love,
Evidence that rich life dwells there.

Don't rush, but stay awhile.
Life is short,
Make your love, long.

— BEVERLY ENGEL

Exercise | **Full Stop**

Often during lovemaking couples get lost in fantasy and lose track of each other. This exercise will help you reestablish the reality that it is the two of you, and only the two of you, who are together now. It will also help you to feel and appreciate the level of arousal you have reached.

1. Some time during lovemaking, one of you can stop all motion, signaling to the other that you want to reconnect emotionally. At first you may want to do this verbally, by saying something like, "Let's stop a minute. I just want to feel you, take you in, to know you are really here with me and I am here with you." Eventually, you may work out a nonverbal signal.

2. Look into each other's eyes and communicate only through your eyes how you are feeling toward each other at the moment.

3. Take in whatever emotions your partner is communicating to you. While it may be difficult, resist the temptation to pull back from any deeper loving feelings your partner is expressing. Take a deep breath, taking in the love, no matter how painful. Feel it deep in your belly and chest. Allow yourself to cry if tears begin to flow.

   If you see fear in your partner's eyes, take this in as well. Take a deep breath and notice whether he is merely reflecting the fear in your own eyes. Acknowledge how frightening it can be to feel so deeply connected, so vulnerable, so deeply loved.

4. Begin to caress each other and take in each other's breath. Acknowledge how grateful you are to have each other. Take at least a minute or two to do this, longer if you wish. If you fall asleep, that's fine. You will awake feeling complete, without any sense of frustration.

   When you have completed the exercise you may feel like hugging each other tightly and communicating how grateful you are for each other's love.

E x e r c i s e | **Time Out**

Time Out is a playful version of Full Stop. You can either set a timer or take turns deciding when to call out "Time Out!" When either the timer goes off or one of you calls "Time Out!" stop all motion completely. Do not move for at least one minute, if not longer. Lie still and be aware of all the sound, smell, taste, and touch sensations you can experience.

When you feel like resuming your lovemaking, breathe in unison as you slowly, tenderly return to the peak of passion. As your breathing increases, so will your motion and your excitement.

Since many of us typically make love in a driven, single-minded way, this exercise will provide valuable distance from that compulsive, edgy feeling and help you let go of your need to perform or reach orgasm. It will also add an element of spontaneity, playfulness, and surprise that is so often missing in routine sex. Finally, it can make love-making more fulfilling when you take time out to appreciate what you are really doing. (Note: both Full Stop and Time Out short-circuit male arousal and thus prolong intercourse indefinitely.)

⑥ Sacred Sexuality ⑥

In the preface to his book *Sacred Sexuality,* Georg Feuerstein defines sacred sexuality as follows.

> *Sacred Sexuality is about love—not merely the positive feeling between inti-*
> *mates but an overwhelming reverence for all embodied life on whatever level*
> *of existence. Through sacred sexuality, we directly participate in the vastness*
> *of being—the mountains, rivers, and animals of the earth, the planets and the*
> *stars, and our next-door neighbors.*

Sacred sexuality is about recovering our authentic being, which knows bliss beyond mere pleasurable sensations. It is a special form of communication, even communion, that fills us with awe and stillness.

Sacred sexuality is about the reenchantment of our lives. It is about embracing the imponderable mystery of existence, about the curious fact that you and I and five billion others cannot account for our existence and our sexuality. [6]

We all have the potential for uplifting experiences of total happiness, when all self-centeredness is suspended and a powerful spiritual force seems to lift us out of ourselves. Those who have had such experiences describe them as "an overwhelming sense of joy" or "a feeling of profound peace."

In this almost mystical state all opposites are transcended, as Self and other are merged into a single whole. There is no within and without, no space and time. Sometimes this kind of breakthrough occurs when we are in love or as a result of sexual intimacy. Indeed, sexual love is the most intense and tangible way in which men and women strive for a union that transcends the boundaries of their everyday experience. It is during the sexual act, more than at any other time, that we seek to merge, to make a deeper connection.

More often than not, this desire remains unconscious, and we engage in sex merely as a diversion from the stresses of daily life. Thus, our sexual contact is only skin-deep and we fail to experience our primal impulse toward union. As a result, we continue to feel alone and unloved on a very deep level.

Tantra and Tantric Sexuality

Tantra has become the most commonly used term to describe consciousness-raising sexual activity. The Sanskrit word *tantra* means "web" and is explained as "that which expands understanding." Tantrism can be defined as a system of beliefs and practices intended to stretch the human mind and to guide it to higher knowledge, or gnosis. Its goal is personal liberation (*mukti*), which is understood as the transcendence of the ego-personality, of ordinary consciousness. This condition is also often referred to as the attainment of unexcelled bliss (*ananda*), or delight.

Tantra is extremely comprehensive and difficult to characterize. Common to all tantric orientations, however, is the idea that the Divine is not separated from creation by an unbridgeable gulf, and that the world is an aspect or manifestation of the Divine.

Tantrism celebrates the divinity in and of every being and thing. Therefore, anything is permissible as long as it leads to the realization of the presence of the Divine here and now. It is in this spirit that some schools of tantrism have also made use of ritualistic sex (*maithuna*).

For many Hindus and Buddhists, tantra is a serious religious path, but tantralike practices are found throughout the world. Native American, Polynesian, Chinese, Egyptian, Scandinavian, and African cultures all have their own versions of tantric sex.

Tantra decrees that sensual joy is to be celebrated but that it is not the end purpose of sex. It is a means through which we can gain a profound realization of the divine nature of existence, epitomized in the sex act. According to tantric beliefs, sex is magnetic because it gives us the sweet taste of higher

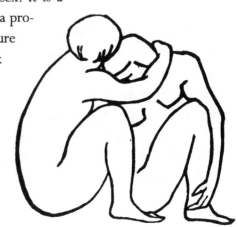

consciousness, of the transcendental, even if it is at first just a flash. Love—self-love and loving others as yourself—is the law of tantra.

Tantric sex is spontaneous, meditative, and intimate lovemaking. Through it you can learn to prolong the act of making love and channel sexual energy instead of dissipating it, thereby raising the level of your consciousness. More important, tantric sex helps you focus on being rather than on doing. There is no goal in tantric sex, only the present moment of perfect and harmonious union.

The aim of tantric sex is to take you out of your head and into your body and your heart, where you will discover your supreme Self hidden deep inside. It is also teaches you to revere your sexual partner and to transform the act of sex into a sacrament of love.

Tantra is also about the lighthearted joy of bodilessness, of formlessness. During your most intense orgasms you have undoubtedly experienced this feeling when you completely lost track of your body, of your partner, even who you are. In tantric sex this feeling of formlessness is expanded and intensified as you become one with your partner and the universe.

Tantra seeks to elevate the sexual act to its highest possible level. In tantric sex the fusion that is felt only briefly during conventional orgasm is experienced consciously and completely, as the individual consciousness unites with cosmic consciousness. Tantra teaches that you cannot transcend sex by denying it. Only the complete, conscious experience of sex can lead to a higher awareness in which a bliss transcending even sexual pleasure is experienced.

The tantric lovemaking techniques that follow can offer you the most exciting and satisfying experiences of your life. Although it is not necessary for you to subscribe to the cultural or spiritual values of traditional tantra, to gain the most from any of these exercises, a person or couple doing them must be sincere about making an effort to go beyond their personal, or limited, self.

Doing this will require you to break some old habits and to change your way of thinking. You will undoubtedly experience some initial resistance, perhaps thinking the exercises foolish or experiencing frustration when your urge to reach orgasm quickly is thwarted. And you may be unhappy about the fact that you are asked to refrain from actual intercourse for two weeks. But once you realize how much this practice helps you go beyond your dependence on physical release and transcend into the realm of loving communion, you will realize it is worth the sacrifice.

Many couples have experienced a profound deepening of their relationship and their erotic life as a result of these tantric experiences. A simple touch, once only experienced as an invitation to intercourse, now expresses a multitude of tender feelings. A kiss opens up an entire universe of pleasure.

Even couples who have been together for many years are able to tap into a power that enables them to experience those feelings of awe and excitement that they shared in the beginning of their relationship. Sexuality becomes fresh and magnetic again.

Tantra and tantric sexuality are very complex traditions. What follows is a brief introduction that will give you just a taste of how you can begin to use some of the tantric techniques to imbue your relationship with more reverence and sacredness. The use of sanskrit terminology is included to further give you the flavor of tantra.

I recommend that those interested in learning more about tantric sexuality refer to the Ramsdale's *Sexual Energy Ecstasy* and other books listed in the Recommended Reading section at the back of the book.

TANTRIC RITUAL

Those who study Buddhist tantra advocate the type of absolute commitment that the average seeker is not willing to make, but Hindu tantrics believe that a sincere, mindful ritual is a sufficient sacrifice for beginners. Ritual constitutes one of the most important aspects of tantra and tantric sex. It will help you to endow each lovemaking experience with special significance and, in so doing, to transform both the experience and yourself.

According to David and Ellen Ramsdale, the authors of *Sexual Energy Ecstasy,* the basic prerequisites for this ritual, sometimes called *samadhi,* are the ability to achieve a degree of meditative calm and an eagerness to experience the spiritual dimension of sex. Both partners should have a mutual goal to attain a higher consciousness, even enlightenment, as opposed to reproduction or erotic pleasure. Beyond that there must be a willingness to embrace the infinite or divine dimension of life.

To begin this process the couple must be able to step beyond their usual view of themselves as man and woman and instead achieve a sense of reverence for each other as god and goddess, as holy beings. The woman is to be worshiped as the perfect expression of divine energy (Shakti) and the man as the ideal expression of divine awareness (Shiva). Together they represent pure consciousness, the perfect, eternal peace and bliss that is our ultimate nature.

HONORING SHAKTI AND SHIVA

In ancient Indian tantric texts the supreme tantric deities are known as Shiva and Shakti. When Shiva, the masculine principle, and his beloved consort, Shakti, the feminine principle, are joined together in sexual union, they are in a blissful state of cosmic consciousness. At this point, there is no division between the god and the goddess, and all sexual duality is dissolved.

In temples throughout India, icons abound symbolizing the harmony of sacred sexual union. The most prevalent and significant of these are the lingam and yoni, often carved from wood or stone. The lingam represents the hallowed phallus of Shiva and is placed within the divine yoni, which represents the vulva of Shakti.

Feminine energy is revered and honored in tantra as the catalyst for sexual and spiritual transformation. According to tantra, Shakti energy is the primal force of nature, and through her the male can transcend his ordinary human condition to attain sexual ecstasy and spiritual realization.

Tantra also teaches a man to honor a woman's sexuality and to surrender himself to its limitless power. He is encouraged to sensually prolong lovemaking so that the woman reaches the height of her sexual joy.

Maithuna

Maithuna, or sexual union, is a ritual sacrifice of body, mind, and self. Ancient tantric belief has it that we descended from light. In this ritual of the five elements, we return to the light. *Maithuna,* symbolizing space, is the culminating stage of the ancient sequence of earth, water, fire, and air. This ritual method follows a gradual approach that progressively refines the senses and uses them as a springboard into illumination.

According to David and Ellen Ramsdale, the various ingredients of the ritual create a recipe that encourages this upward progress of energy.

> *Incense and perfume appeal to the sense of smell, stimulating the root energy center in the cervix or perineum. Wine and other liquid refreshment arouse taste awareness at the sex center in the lower belly. The sight of the beloved and the dancing fire of the ritual candles awaken the solar plexus. The practice of nyasa as well as other forms of touching during the ceremony activate the heart. Sounds, such as ritual music and the mantras that you repeat together, stimulate the throat center. At the top of this sensual ladder of ritual love lies the third eye, linked to the core of the brain. The kiss of your undivided attention will wake it up.* [7]

PREPARATIONS

The sacredness and purity of the environment in which you perform your tantric rituals is very important. It is believed that by creating a harmonious environment you can establish an inner state of tranquillity and equilibrium. In traditional tantric texts there are precise and detailed instructions on how to set up hallowed places of worship, but you can create a sanctuary in your home that reflects your own beliefs and lifestyle. The most important criteria for your sacred space is that it be clean, uncluttered, and undisturbed by outside interference.

If you have already created your sensual refuge, you're one step ahead. You may want to add any or all of the following items.

❖ *Introduce the tantric colors of reds, oranges, purples, and gold, colors that stimulate the chakras, awaken the senses, and ignite sexual energy. Muslin, traditional Indian saris, and exotic textiles can disguise furniture and other objects that can't be removed from the room.*

❖ *Create an altar to remind you that your acts are dedicated to love and consciousness. Your tantric altar can be as simple or elaborate as you wish to make it, but the objects placed on it should have special significance to you. Traditional offerings include incense, ritual foods, fresh and fragrant flowers, and you should always place a lighted candle on your altar during rituals.*

❖ *On the floor or other suitable surface, you may want to draw a large mandala consisting of two triangles interwoven within a circle. One should be pointed up, the other down. This is an ancient symbol of integration.*

Before beginning follow these instructions:

❖ *Always begin by lighting a candle and purifying the environment using sage or incense, preferably sandlewood.*

❖ *Purify your bodies to transform them into temples of consciousness. Ritually bathe each other, allowing the warm water to cascade over your bodies to wash away all external and internal impurities.*

❖ *Anoint each other with essential oils such as rose, jasmine, and patchouli on the palms, feet, third eyes, eyelids, earlobes, lips, breasts, navels, and genitals. Known as* nyasa, *this can be performed either in silent reverence or while repeating the Sanskrit holy word "Om," or "you are my god / goddess" as you anoint each body part.*

❖ *Physical purification is followed by mental purification. After meditat-*
ing using a mantra such as "Om" or "God is love," contemplate the
unity of cosmic male and female represented by the symbol of triangles
interlaced within the circle.

❖ *Take turns worshiping each other's bodies, revering them as a physical*
manifestation of the god or goddess. Kneel before your partner. Perceive
her or him to be the sacred embodiment of the goddess Shakti or the
god Shiva. Touch and honor each part of your partner's body so that
your every touch and kiss is filled with love. The man should then
scatter fragrant petals onto the woman's yoni, revering it as the sacred
gateway to sexual ecstasy. Then the woman can perform a similar rit-
ual, touching her lover's body with deep veneration and spiritual
devotion, scattering scented petals over his lingam.

THE TANTRIC KISS

Although the tantric kiss awakens erotic responses in the entire body and
ignites flames of passion, it is not a prelude to further sexual activity, nor
should it have any specific goal. Instead, it is a profoundly intimate sexual
exchange between two lovers that should be valued for what it is—a peak
experience of timelessness and merging. In tantra, it is said that the
exchange of body fluids, which occurs in deep and intimate kissing, har-
monizes and balances male and female cosmic energies. Lovers' mouths
symbolize the divine union of the tantric deities: the soft yielding of the lips
is like the softness of the female yoni, and the penetrative action of the
tongue corresponds to the penetration of the male lingam.

Never rush into a full penetrative kiss, but begin by placing small tender kisses along your lover's upper and lower lips. Run the tip of your
tongue sensuously over their moist softness. Let your mouths and tongues
gently play and seek a balance between active and passive roles. Finally, lose
yourselves in a deep tantric kiss and allow your physical and emotional
boundaries to dissolve in the warm, full contact of your lips.

BLISSFUL UNION

Sit in front of each other and breathe together so that your inhales and exhales are of the same duration. Remain mindful of balancing your breath in this way throughout the ritual. You may chant "Om" together on the exhalation if you wish. Concentrate your mind on the *muladhara,* or root, chakra at the cervix, perineum, or at the base of the spine.

After a while you will begin to experience an energy rising up your back. Consciously draw this energy up the spine with each inhalation and then give this energy to your partner with the exhalation.

When this energy is very strong, the male partner draws the female partner to him. Lingam and yoni are briefly worshiped. She sits in his lap in the classic position, called *yabyum,* and brings his lingam into her yoni. (To achieve this position, face each other sitting cross-legged on the floor. The woman then rises up and sits on the male's legs, wrapping her legs around his waist so that her yoni is connecting with his lingam. You can also achieve *yabyum* from the missionary position by embracing each other and allowing the male to pull you both up in a sitting position or from female dominant positions.) Remaining completely motionless, begin the sex meditation.

When the woman sits on top of the man in tantric sex it is not so she can imitate the man and become aggressive. The yabyum position enables the woman to set the pace until the couple begins to move in unision. It also helps to inhibit the man's tendency to move rapidly since he cannot do so as readily in this position. Also, in this position if the man's erection subsides the penis cannot slip out.

Do not plan what you are going to do but let the life force take over. Then surrender to it and it becomes a meditation, allowing you to enjoy the here and now more completely. The body has its own wisdom and moves accordingly.

Do not hurry, and do not push for the end. Through tantra a deep silent communion occurs between two body energies and then you can remain together for hours if you wish.

Your eyes and mental focus should be on your partner's third eye, the space between and just above the eyebrows. Continuing your breath awareness, bring your foreheads together and join your eyes into one. Even though this may seem awkward at first, it quickly leads to a fusion of consciousness.

It is important to stay with this merging of the eyes. It keeps the mind alert, preventing daydreaming, sleepiness, and self-consciousness. By keeping your attention firmly on the third eye, you will avoid the usual pull toward genital stimulation.

The desire for sex is actually a desire for *oneness*. Through tantra you and your partner can find that oneness if you are willing to surrender.

Tantra is the path of surrender. It asks that you float with the stream of life, not against it. The mind is no longer in the way, and your hearts beat as one.

According to the Ramsdales, while this kind of meditation for the attainment of higher consciousness is not unique to India or to Hindu tantra yoga, this particular technique, also called *lata sadhana,* has been tried and tested over the centuries. Demanding as this practice is, when a couple does succeed in experiencing total fusion, their relationship will be forever elevated to a higher, more fulfilling plane.

Though obviously not for everyone, in this discipline lies the total fulfillment implied by the primal gesture toward union that we call sex. Those interested in the yoga training behind the method may want to explore the tantra yoga system.

AFTERGLOW

The moments following sexual union can be very precious if you are both able to treasure the stillness and sense of merging. Do not rush away from your sacred space but relax totally and bask in the afterglow. According to tantric teachings, it is then that the energies can fuse and find a state of equilibrium so that you feel refreshed and replenished.

The emphasis on sex in our society is an attempt to fill a vast emptiness. In our heart of hearts, all we really want is unconditional love. When sex is offered as a gift, as an expression of unconditional love, it becomes the great gift of life itself.

By practicing the exercises in this chapter you will open yourself up to a whole new range of sexual experiences. As you continue to learn how to reach the heights of ecstasy together, you will also learn the secrets of true intimacy. As your joy multiplies, your relationship and your love will grow deeper and stronger.

Part III

❖ ❖ ❖

The Four Seasons of Sensuous Passion

Sex is discovery.

— FANNIE HURST

Knowing is the most profound

kind of love, giving someone

the gift of knowledge about yourself.

— MARSHA NORMAN

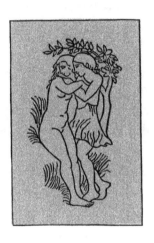

Springtime:
The First Stages
of Passion

The beginning of a love affair has often been likened to springtime, a time of discovery, blossoming, anticipation of wonderful things to come, a time of birth and rebirth. If you are just beginning a relationship or are just recently married, this chapter will help you to make the most of this magical time.

As you have read in the first part of this book, sensuality is a key factor in maintaining a vital, exciting, and fulfilling sexual relationship. For this reason I encourage you as new lovers to take the time to explore each other's bodies using all your senses. If you do this you will be rewarded for years to come.

Fortunately, when we first fall in love we want to get to know every inch of our loved one's body. It is during this time more than any other that lovers are willing to spend hours discovering every nook and cranny, falling in love with everything that makes their lover unique, from the way their little toe bends, to those precious little dimples on their behind. If this is the case with you, the following exercises will simply reinforce this tendency and offer you ideas for how to continue your explorations.

E x e r c i s e | **Exploring with Your Eyes Closed**

By deliberately blocking out one of our senses, we can intensify our awareness of the other senses. The following exercise will help you to discover your partner on an entirely new level.

1. Ask your partner to lie down, face down to begin with. Explain that you will be touching with your eyes closed and encourage him to do the same as you explore his body. Encourage him to relax into the situation, putting all embarrassment or self-judgment aside.

2. Slowly begin to explore your partner's body with your eyes completely closed. Imagine that you are blind and just meeting your partner for the first time and want to get to know how he looks by using your fingertips. You may feel awkward at first, but you will soon get into it.

Having your eyes closed will force you to rely on your senses of touch, taste, and smell—rather than your vision—to discover your partner's body. It also will force you to go slowly. It will cause you to notice things about his body that you never noticed before, such as variations in the softness of his skin and how various parts of his body smell and taste. You may also be able to reach a level of intimacy that few other experiences can provide.

Exercise | **No Hands**

We generally depend on our hands to pleasure and explore our partner's body, but we could use our entire body. In this exercise you will caress your partner using your entire body—your torso, your arms, your legs, your face, and your mouth. If you are limber enough, you can even use your buttocks. Just don't use your hands.

1. Have your partner lie down on her stomach to begin. Spread oil on both your body and your partner's body, making sure to cover the entire surface.

2. Now let your imagination run wild. Start wherever you like, with your partner's feet or with her shoulders, but move up and down her body systematically, not randomly. Take plenty of time with each part of her body. Remember, your intention is to get to know your partner's body and to communicate the love you feel. Here are some suggestions:

❖ *Starting with her shoulders, use your forearm to trace the curve of her shoulders down to her arms and hands.*

❖ *Place your chest against her back and move around, feeling the smoothness of her skin against your own. Do the same with her buttocks and notice how much softer the skin is in this area.*

❖ *Put oil on the side of your face and explore your partner's back and buttocks using only your face. (Caution: some men may have coarse stubble on their face that could cause their partner pain or irritation. If this your situation, be sure to shave first or use a different part of your body.)*

❖ *Caress your partner's legs using your legs.*

❖ *Explore your partner's feet, legs, buttocks, and back using only your feet. Be creative: use the bottoms of your feet, your arches, and your toes to sensuously titillate your partner.*

❖ *Oil your buttocks and gently slide them over your partner's buttocks.*

❖ *Have your partner turn over, and using your oiled chest only, explore the front of her body—her chest, stomach, and pelvic area.*

Exercise | Mouth Only

This exercise is a variation on the one above and has infinite possibilities. It offers a unique way to get to know your partner's body and is also an exciting way to express your love and ignite passion in your lover. And since there are more nerve endings in our lips than in most other parts of the body, there is a good chance it will fire your passion as well.

Preparation: If you are worried about taste or smell, take a sensual shower together beforehand.

1. Begin exploring your partner's body using only your mouth. Starting at your partner's head, use your lips and tongue to kiss, lick, suck, and gently nibble her entire body, all the way down to her feet. Notice the various textures of her body against your lips—the smoothness of her forehead, the softness of her stomach, the roughness of her elbows. Pay attention to the fact that her body temperature will vary depending on which part of her body you are exploring. Using your tongue, notice the different tastes of different parts—from salty to sweet, from bland to pungent.

2. Ask your partner to turn over, and continue your explorations with the front of her body. Give yourself permission to be more creative and venture into uncharted territory. There's no telling where your explorations will lead you!

⑥ Communication as Discovery ⑥

In addition to getting to know how your lover's body looks and feels, you will also want to know how to please him sexually and sensually. This includes wanting to know his likes and dislikes, what type of touch he prefers, and how he can best reach orgasm. Unfortunately, some new couples are so caught up in their passion for each other that they don't take the time to communicate these things. During the first stages of passion or the "honeymoon" phase of a relationship partners often tend to focus on trying to please each other more than on being honest about their real desires, preferences, and needs. Moreover, many people are not completely clear about what their own sexual preferences and needs are.

It is important to open the communication early on in a new relationship. Because of your lack of familiarity with each other, it is even more important to share specific information early on. Letting your partner know what you like and don't like sexually in the beginning of a relationship helps to prevent negative patterns from developing.

People in new relationships usually make love to their new partner by doing what turns them on, by doing what pleased a previous partner, or by doing what they have read women or men like. During the honeymoon period everything tends to feel good, but people become more discriminating as time goes by. At that point, if you don't let your partner know what turns you on or off, you will only reinforce the belief that what is being done is okay, thus encouraging your partner to continue as they have.

There are two basic methods of communicating sexual information to your partner—nonverbally, through the use of body movements during lovemaking, or verbally, by talking with your lover either during lovemaking or at some other time. Both methods have advantages and disadvantages.

You may find that talking during lovemaking spoils the mood for you, so you prefer to rely on body movements and sounds of pleasure. Or, conversely, you may find that talking about sex while you are making love enhances the experience for you. Some people find it extremely arousing to talk to their partner about what they want to do to her or him. What is important is that you develop some form of communication that is comfortable for you and your partner, whether it is verbal or nonverbal.

⑥   Nonverbal Communication   ⑨

Nonverbal communication can often be more precise than verbal communication. For example, many women need very specific clitoral stimulation in order to reach orgasm. Attempting to describe the type of stimulation needed can be difficult, if not impossible. However, directing your partner nonverbally, by actually taking his hand in yours and moving it in the desired manner can communicate your needs very effectively.

The following three exercises will slow you down during lovemaking and help you focus on sensual touch and sensual pleasures. This, in turn, will help each of you identify the kinds of touch you like to give and receive. The exercises also (perhaps most important) provide a way to communicate these preference to each other. They will be especially beneficial to those of you who have difficulty verbalizing your sexual needs, preferences, and desires. They will show you a way to communicate with your partner just by moving your hands to the places where you like to be touched and also show you a way to direct your partner in the type of touch you prefer.

Exercise | **The Face Caress**

The face caress is part of the sensate focus program I have already introduced you to. It is designed to establish warm, positive, effective nonverbal communication between partners.

Preparation: You will need a clock, a large beach towel and a bath towel, a pillow, and massage oil. Choose an oil that you and your partner both like, one that will not irritate your skin. Some people do not like oil of any kind on their face, but a light lotion can work almost as well. Try to stay away from anything that is heavily scented, because you will be applying the oil close to the nose, and you don't want the scent to be distracting. Vitamin E or aloe vera cream both work well.

Wear comfortable, loose clothes such as T-shirts and shorts. Females may wish to wear a halter top. This exercise is done most comfortably on a bed, but you can also use a futon or spread a beach towel on the floor.

1. The active partner should sit with her back against the headboard of the bed or against a wall with a pillow on her lap. The passive partner should lie face up, between the active partner's legs, head on the pillow. Make sure the passive partner's face is within easy reach.

2. The face caress includes the face, ears, sides of the neck, shoulders, and the top of the chest. As the active partner, you will begin by warming some oil or lotion in your hand. Then begin to caress your partner's face, starting with his forehead. Remember that caressing is an extremely slow, sensuous touch. Slowly and gently glide either one or both of your hands across the full length of the forehead several times using the flat of your fingers, your palms, and your wrist.

3. Lightly caress his eyebrows with the flat of your fingers, as well as the eyelids and underneath the eyes.

4. Gently caress the bridge and the sides of the nose very briefly.

5. Now move down to the cheeks. Experiment with a variety of strokes. For example, begin by gently cupping his cheeks in your hands. Then start at the outer edges of the nose and gently move out toward the ears. Briefly use a circular motion using your palms. Or make long, sweeping motions starting at the chin and moving up the entire side of the face, using the flat of your fingers, your palms, and wrist.

6. Now move to his ears. Begin by cupping them gently in your palms. Now stroke the outer edges of the ears with the flat of your fingers. Using the tips of your fingers, gently stroke the inside ridges, making sure you do not enter the ear itself. Finish by gently stroking his earlobes.

7. Gently move across his chin and along the jawline using your palms.

8. Move down the sides of the neck and then back up using long strokes (never move across it or put any pressure whatsoever under the chin, because this can evoke a strangling sensation in many people).

9. Finally, move down to his shoulders and the very top of the chest, again using sweeping motions. Do not proceed to the breasts.
    Continue this caress for fifteen minutes. When you have finished, slowly remove your hands and allow the passive partner to remain quiet for a few minutes. Do not talk or ask for feedback.

10. Ask your partner to place his hands on top of yours and to direct you to the areas of his face, neck, and shoulders that he liked having touched the most. Then ask him to show you which type of touch he preferred by guiding your hands in these motions.

11. Now spend a few minutes touching this part of his body in the way that your partner has directed you.

Switch roles, with you now being the passive person.

After you have completed the exercise, feel free to give each other feedback. Be sure to answer the following questions.

❖ *How did you like having your face caressed?*

❖ *Was there any part of the exercise that was uncomfortable? Caressing the face can cause a person to feel very vulnerable and a little like their privacy is being invaded, or it can create a deep sense of knowing that you are loved. Did you feel either way, or was your experience entirely different?*

❖ *Were you able to communicate your preferences to your partner by guiding her hand?*

❖ *Was your partner able to nonverbally communicate to you what he preferred?*

  If you or your partner were unable to adequately communicate nonverbally the kind of touch you each preferred, tell her verbally and then have your partner try it again until she gets it just right.

E x e r c i s e | **Showing Your Partner What You Like**

This exercise will take courage, but the benefits are so numerous that it is well worth it. You are essentially going to show your partner how you like to be touched. This exercise is especially beneficial for women, who may require a softer touch than their partner might normally give.

1. Begin by slowly caressing what are considered the less sexual parts of your own body while your partner watches. Caress your shoulders, your arms, your hands. Touch yourself in the way that feels best to you, using oil if you wish. Do this exercise without speaking, but feel free to make sounds of pleasure if you wish.

2. Continue on to your chest, then your stomach, and finally your hips. Allow yourself to really get into the touching. Close your eyes if this will help you to be less self-conscious.

3. Now move to your feet, your calves, and finally, your thighs.

4. Show your lover what you like, what excites you the most as you move in closer to your genitals. Open your eyes if you'd like to see the excitement on your lover's face as you begin to touch your genitals, or keep them closed if this helps you get into the sensations.

5. If you aren't too self-conscious, show your lover the kinds of touch you need to reach orgasm. Know without any doubt that your partner is enjoying watching you and remember that this is one of the best ways for you to communicate your preferences. As your partner watches you become more and more excited, he will remember what kind of touch turns you on and will be eager to bring you to this level of excitement the next time.

   If you feel too self-conscious to do this exercise comfortably, show your partner how you like to be sexually pleasured by placing your hand gently on top of his and guiding him in terms of firmness and speed.

Exercise | The Genital Caress

The genital caress is another sensate focus exercise developed by Masters and Johnson to help couples connect with one another on a more sensuous level. It will help you to continue exploring each other's bodies and to communicate nonverbally about your likes and dislikes. It will also help if either one of you has issues with your body image, particularly if you have concerns about the size or shape of your genitals. By recognizing that your partner can find pleasure in touching your genitals and by learning to take pleasure in it yourself, you will learn to accept those parts of your body better.

Preparations: Before beginning this exercise, make sure you have at least an hour to an hour and a half of uninterrupted time. Once again, you will need a quiet room that is conducive to relaxation and sensuality. You will also need a towel, a natural-based massage oil, and a lubricant like K-Y jelly or Physicians Formula Emollient Oil to use as a genital lubricant. Jojoba, which is too viscous to use for body massage, is delightful for genital lubrication.

Before beginning this exercise, do some spoon breathing to help you relax and connect, and give each other a short full-body caress.

During the first part of the exercise, agree that there will be no talking unless one of you becomes uncomfortable.

When you are the passive person, place your arms at your sides, palms up. Close your eyes, take some deep breaths, and remember to breathe throughout the exercise. If you feel your muscles tensing, breathe and try to relax your stomach, leg, and buttock muscles. As you receive the caress, all you need to do is focus on your own sensations.

The Position: When the male is the receiver he will lie flat on his back and position himself so that his legs are over his partner's legs. The female will sit up in bed with her back leaning against the headboard or wall, with her legs underneath her partner's legs. Thus his genitals are in her lap and she can easily reach and caress his penis, testicles, lower abdomen, and chest.

When the female is the receiver, she will lie on her back on the bed resting her legs on her partner's legs as he sits with his back against the wall or headboard with legs stretched out. Her legs are thus open with her vulva exposed. This position, called a nondemand position, is very beneficial in stimulating areas of the vagina that the female has identified as feeling particularly pleasurable.

Now you are ready to begin. The active partner pours some oil into the palm of his or her hand, and beginning at the lower part of the thighs, begins to gently caress the outside of the thighs using long, slow strokes. Move on to the tops of the thighs and then to the inner thighs. Remember to use the flat of your fingers, your palm, your wrist, and your forearm rather than your fingertips.

If you are a male in the active role, caress the front of your partner's body for about ten minutes and then warm some lubricant in your hand and slowly move your fingers over your partner's outer vaginal lips. You will be caressing for your own pleasure, taking your time to explore and notice the different textures and temperatures. Now move on to the inner lips. Finally, move on to the clitoris. Don't rub her clitoris, caress it slowly. Your purpose is not to turn her on but to pleasure her and yourself. Now slowly, very slowly, insert your finger inside her vagina, making sure you use plenty of lubricant. Pay attention to how it feels inside. Feel the vaginal walls and the muscles around the vaginal opening. Think of the inside of the vagina as a clock, and move your fingers in a circle starting and ending at twelve o'clock. Take this opportunity to learn how your partner's genitals feel. Don't slip into trying to turn her on.

If you are a female in the active role, after caressing the front of your partner's body for about ten minutes using lots of lubrication, begin slowly to caress his penis and scrotum with the flat of your fingers and with your palm and wrist. Remember that you are doing this not to turn him on but for your own enjoyment and to learn what your partner's genitals look and feel like.

Slowly move your fingers and hand around the shaft and head of his penis, then slowly run your fingers around each testicle. Experience what the skin feels like on the different areas of the genitals. Notice the different textures and temperatures.

It doesn't matter whether or not your partner has an erection during this exercise. Your purpose is not to arouse him. If he becomes aroused and ejaculates, that's okay. Gently wipe him off and continue the caress. Do the genital caress for at least fifteen minutes.

❖ *Always complete the exercise by gradually moving away from the genitals toward the inner thighs and finally upward to the outer thighs.*

❖ *After you have completed the caress, have the passive partner give feedback about what she liked and disliked. Have your partner* describe one or two things that she especially enjoyed. Now do the caress again, incorporating what your partner has told you. Ask your partner for more feedback. Do the caress until she feels that you are doing it just right.

❖ Ask your partner if there was something you didn't do that he would have liked. Ask him to give you explicit instructions on how to administer this touch, and then try it, asking for feedback as you go along. If you are still unable to give your partner what he desires, ask him to guide you with his hand until you get it right.

⑥ Verbal Communication ⑥

Many people believe that their partners should be sensitive enough to know their needs without even being told. How often have you heard someone say, "If I have to ask for it, I don't want it." When you think about it, doesn't this seem rather silly? Don't allow this kind of misguided thinking to get in the way of your receiving the kind of touching and stimulation that you really desire. Remember, no one is a mind reader, and no matter how well your partner knows you, there is really no way for her to know what you want sexually at any given time.

Some people are afraid to ask for what they want sexually for fear of being rejected. If they are able to ask at all, they couch their requests in indirect language, hoping their wishes will be understood but protecting themselves in case they're not. Unfortunately, the fear of not getting what they want can create a self-fulfilling prophecy. If you don't ask for what you want directly, your partner may never know what you really desire. And if you interpret not getting what you want as a confirmation that you were right not to ask because you wouldn't have gotten what you wanted anyway, then you won't make your needs known the next time, either. Although it is difficult, being vulnerable with your partner by openly communicating your sexual preferences is an excellent way of building trust with your partner.

Many people also have the erroneous belief that the best way to communicate their desires to their partner is to do to their partner what they would like their partner to do to them. Unfortunately, this method of communication leaves just too much room for miscommunication. The main drawback to nonverbal communication is that it can be misunderstood. Often verbal communication is necessary to straighten out the confusion created by nonverbal communication.

In a survey conducted by Philip and Lorna Sarrel, sex therapists at Yale University, it was found that among women who have told their partners exactly how they like to be touched, seven out of ten indicated they have orgasms "every time" or "almost every time" they make love. The Sarrels concluded that the ability to share thoughts and feelings about sex with your partner is the single most important factor in a good sexual relationship. They also found that the good communicators had intercourse more often and were more likely to be satisfied with its frequency.

Many sex experts feel that the best time to talk about sexual matters is not when you're ready to have sex, or during sex, but at some other time. Then you and your partner will both be less likely to perceive suggestions and information as criticism.

The following suggestions will help you communicate with each other and discover your desires, preferences, and needs, first on a less threatening level and then on a sexual level.

❖ *Start by sharing your favorite tactile experiences (lying on a warm beach, walking in the rain, taking a long bath, receiving a massage) and your favorite textures (satin, silk, cotton, wool).*

❖ *Tell your partner what part of your body is your favorite and what part you like to have touched the most (they may or may not be the same).*

❖ *Talk about the part of your partner's body that you like the most and the part that you like to touch the most. If you aren't sure what this is, do some experimenting.*

❖ *Share your favorite sexual experience together. Tell your partner what it was about this particular experience that was thrilling and/or fulfilling.*

❖ *Tell each other one thing you wish your partner would do more often or do differently sexually.*

⑥ Discovering Your Partner's Erogenous Zones ⑥

There are many erogenous zones, or "hot spots," besides the genitals. Not everyone is sensitive in the same way, but generally speaking these areas are:

❖ *The lips, which respond not only to kissing but to gentle touching with the fingers, licking, sucking, and even nibbling.*

❖ *The eyelids, which respond to a gentle brush of the fingertips or tongue.*

❖ *The area between the eyebrows, which responds to a gentle rub or lick.*

❖ *The ears, which respond to warm breath and having the tongue inserted. The earlobes can also be licked, sucked, or nibbled.*

❖ *The nape of the neck, which responds to blowing, kissing, and licking.*

❖ *The middle of the palm, which responds when a middle finger is pressed into it and rotated in little circles.*

❖ *The little finger, which responds to caressing, licking, and sucking, especially along the outer edge.*

❖ *The nipples, on both men and women, respond to sucking, licking, gentle tugging, and nibbling.*

❖ *The armpits, especially in women, can elicit sexual feelings when they are gently bitten or when a penis is inserted there.*

❖ *The area between the breasts is an erotic zone for men and women. Lightly caressing or licking the entire valley between the breasts can be quite stimulating.*

❖ *The navel responds to a tongue inside going in small circles.*

❖ *The base of the spine can elicit deep sexual feelings when warmed by a hand stroking in circles.*

❖ *The buttocks respond to caressing, tickling, licking, and sucking, but they can also respond to light slapping and deep probing.*

❖ *The insides of the thighs respond to light touching and licking.*

❖ *The knees respond to light touch and licking, as does the hollow behind the knees.*

❖ *The feet, particularly the toes, respond to licking and sucking. Sucking the big toe can be especially arousing.*

❖ *The anus is a powerful erotic zone when a finger is inserted at the peak of genital orgasm.*

An important part of getting to know your partner sexually is learning what parts of her body arouse the most passionate feelings in her. Try tickling, caressing, stroking, and kissing all these parts and asking your partner for her reaction. Sometimes stimulating any of these areas may actually be irritating, so feedback is essential.

After you have learned your partner's erogenous zones, encourage him to explore yours. We don't always know whether something feels good until someone actually stimulates these areas. Be sure to be specific about what you like and don't like. For example, you may not like it when your partner puts his tongue in your ear, but when he nibbles on your earlobe it may send you through the ceiling.

☺ Learning How to Pleasure Your Lover Orally ☺

Many new couples have difficulties with oral sex. Both men and women are often squeamish about it, sometimes because of concerns about smell or hygiene, and sometimes because of lack of experience. Ironically, as much as they might resist giving oral sex to their partner, most people desire having their partner give oral sex to them. This obviously poses a problem. Those who are unable to give oral sex are obviously reluctant to ask for it because no one wants to be perceived as selfish. Therefore, neither partner asks and they both end up not getting their needs met.

Many people, men and women, desire oral sex, since it is one of the most highly sensuous and erotic sex acts. Rightly or wrongly, both sexes tend to experience oral sex as proof that their partner loves them and accepts their body totally. Many women cannot have an orgasm with intercourse, but they can with oral sex. And there is, perhaps, no greater thrill for a man than to see and feel his partner enthusiastically loving his penis.

If you are concerned about hygiene or smell, taking a shower or bath together before making love can help. Or you can incorporate washing your partner's genitals into your sensual play. Mildly scented liquid soap, such as Dr. Bronner's, works especially well for this purpose.

The key to satisfying oral sex is to go slowly and to get into the pleasure of the experience, instead of trying to make your partner have an orgasm quickly.

The following sections offer some guidance on how to pleasure your partner orally in a way that provides optimum enjoyment for both the giver and receiver. You may do this silently, asking your partner to tell you only if something is uncomfortable, or you may wish to communicate throughout, especially the first time you try, asking whether what you are doing is pleasurable or whether your partner would like you to do something harder or softer, faster or slower.

Pleasuring the Penis

If you have never given oral sex to a man, the following suggestions may help you feel less self-conscious and more secure about what you are doing. I would like to stress that these are suggestions. It is far more important that you focus on doing what feels good to you and that you begin with an attitude of openness to discovering what brings pleasure to both of you.

Position yourself so that you are facing your partner, preferably with him lying down. In this position the most sensitive areas of the penis—the tip, the frenulum, the crown, and the notch beneath it—are all presented to you. Find a position that is comfortable for you, either lying or sitting at his side or on your knees positioned between his legs.

❖ *Start by massaging his inner thighs, stroking up his inner thighs, and then down the top of his thighs. Teasingly kiss and lick his upper thighs.*

❖ *Try communicating your love and acceptance by giving your partner gentle kisses all around his genital area.*

❖ *Gently pull on the scrotum, and, if you like, put his balls in your mouth. Pull down gently with your mouth, making sure to avoid pulling on his pubic hair.*

❖ *Place your fingers so that they are poised around his shaft as if to play a musical instrument. Lick your lips to moisten them before you begin.*

❖ *Many men like downward strokes, so begin stroking the penis with your tongue, from the head down to the base. Notice the texture against your tongue.*

❖ *Take your tongue and roll it around the corona (the ridge around the head of the penis). Notice the difference in the texture. Work your tongue gently down the shaft and back up.*

❖ *Flick your tongue in and around the corona and the top of the penis as if you were licking an ice cream cone. Do a series of fast*

licks, and then gently breathe out to tantalize him. Take a break
from stimulating the corona and slide your tongue gently up and
down the shaft.

❖ *Mixing oral sex with manual stimulation can provide a break for you
and can be very exciting for your partner. Since some men will want
lubrication, a little saliva on your index finger may be enough, or you
may want to use sensual jojoba oil or a vegetable oil mix. Begin by
circling your lubricated finger around the corona, then place your
hand below the corona and do quick squeezes down the shaft.
Alternate with a sliding squeeze that finishes with pulling his balls
down a little.*

❖ *Twirl your tongue around the corona, firmly surrounding it with your
lips. Move your tongue along the side and up and down. Intersperse
this with massaging his balls and pulling them down a little.*

❖ *Quickly give feather strokes with your hands on the shaft, continuing
down over and past his balls and onto his thighs, all the while
twirling your tongue around the corona. Do an occasional hard suck
from the corona up.*

❖ *If you feel like it, try the deep suck made famous by the movie* Deep
Throat. *Go very gradually and teasingly. Take at least a full minute
to take his penis as far down your throat as you can. Relax the back of
your throat as much as possible. You may not be able to take his penis
very far down at all the first time you try it. People have a natural
gag response, and some women begin to feel panicky. If this happens,
incorporate your need for a break with teasing your partner. Go back
up to the corona and start all over again. (You can practice relaxing
the muscles at the back of your throat with a cucumber or dildo. It
helps if you continue swallowing.)*

It is important to let your partner know that you would prefer him not to
move his penis around vigorously when it is in your mouth. This only makes
your task more difficult and could cause either or both of you pain.

If you choose to swallow his ejaculate, try to hold his penis as deeply in your mouth as possible. Most men prefer this, since they shrink as they ejaculate. Flick your tongue back and forth at the tip to make it more arousing. If your hand is well lubricated, he may like for you to rub on the shaft as he comes.

The taste of semen varies depending on a man's diet and health. If you don't want to taste it, keep the back of your mouth open and it will not go over your tongue.

Of course, you may not choose to swallow the ejaculate at all, and this is perfectly fine. In fact, if you have any worries about STDs, it is much safer not to. Instead, keep a towel or tissue handy.

One safe-sex strategy is to lubricate the penis with a drop or two of water-based oil and to slip a condom over it. Then stimulate his penis by moving the condom up, down, and around. If you want to switch to intercourse, discard the condom, dry off his penis, and apply a new condom lubricated on the outside.

Pleasuring the Vagina

It is surprising how many men, even with all the information available these days, don't know how to please their partner orally. Many men view their lover's genitals as a puzzle, especially when it comes to oral sex. They feel lost, as if in a maze, and wander around hoping to find a magical answer to the question of what they're doing there.

If this is how you feel, the following instructions will help you immensely. But even more important than following instructions is changing your attitude. Many men perceive the vagina as dirty and oral sex as something to be avoided if at all possible. Or they view oral sex as a chore to be performed in order to get their partner to give them oral sex or as a way of readying their partner for intercourse.

But in the East, particularly in the sacred sex traditions of India, the vagina, or yoni, was viewed as a sacred flower. You have no doubt seen pictures of vaginas drawn as flowers, with the woman's labia drawn as the outer petals. If you can begin to think of your lover's vagina in this way, it will enhance both her pleasure and yours.

Viewing the woman's genitals as a flower will remind you of how sensitive they are. To properly arouse most women, it is best to start at the periphery of the body and gradually move in toward the center of the body, leaving the genitals and especially the clitoris for last. For example, in Taoist sexology, the man arouses the woman by first rubbing her hands and feet, then gradually massaging her up her legs, down her arms to her belly, and eventually to her genitals.

❖ *Position yourself so that your lover's vagina is facing you. Begin stimulating her breasts, including her nipples, with your hands and eventually with your mouth. Now move your hands down to her navel, making a circle with your hands. Move your mouth from between her breasts to her navel. Circle her navel with your tongue, and begin playing with her pubic hair and pubic mound with your hands. Now move your mouth slowly from her navel to her pubic mound. Exhale, allowing your breath to warm and tease her.*

❖ *Begin making several long strokes with your hands up and down her thighs. Notice the smoothness of her thighs and how much smoother her inner thighs are. Some women like their partner to move his hands up to stimulate her breasts and nipples from time to time. Try doing this, and notice how she responds.*

❖ *Now kiss and lick all the way down her inner thigh to the soft hollow behind her knees. Repeat on her other thigh. Now move your mouth up each leg.*

❖ *As you look at your partner's vagina, you will notice that it is surrounded by outer and inner lips. Using a lubricant (your saliva is preferable at this point), slowly begin to stroke her outer lips. Do this until her inner lips begin to open on their own.*

❖ *Now do the same using your mouth. Trace the outline of her outer lips, then her inner lips. Now slowly insert you tongue into the vaginal opening, penetrating as you would with your penis.*

In Eastern erotic writing, orally loving a woman is often compared to the relationship between the bee and the lotus flower. Because of the excitement provoked by the bee's activities deep in the lotus, the flower eventually climaxes, secreting nectarlike substances of nourishing sweetness. In these writings, the fluids that the woman secretes as she becomes aroused and, especially, as she orgasms are considered the nectar of the goddess. These fluids, imbibed orally or absorbed by the penis through osmosis during intercourse immediately after oral love, are considered highly beneficial to male well-being. The Taoists share this idea.

As you allow your tongue to slowly penetrate to the center of your lover's flower, take in her nourishing nectar, allow it to feed your body and soul.

❖ *Now slowly open her petals with your fingers and using your lips and tongue, go from the bottom of her vagina up in the direction of her clitoris. Suck as you nibble. You can move your head from side to side or up and down to provide added stimulation. From time to time, insert your tongue into her vagina and search for her nectar.*

❖ *Try placing your mouth on her pubic mound just where the clitoris begins, and use your fingers or tongue to push the hood of her clitoris back. Applying pressure with your hands on both sides helps to lift her clitoris up and further expose it.*

❖ *Women like various types of clitoral stimulation, but one of the best is to place your lips around the clitoris as you suck and lick with your tongue. Some women prefer mostly sucking with some movement of your head back and forth, while others prefer mostly licking, either slowly and gently or fast and hard. Pay attention to any movement of her body that may give you an indication of what she prefers. (The ideal is for you to devise a nonverbal system ahead of time or for her to direct you verbally as you go.) The important thing is that once you have planted your mouth firmly, do not take it away. Stay in place, but gradually increase the stimulation.*

❖ *Add to her excitement by stimulating her buttocks and inner thighs with your hands or by inserting one or two fingers into her vagina.*

❖ *As they approach orgasm, most women require that the oral loving become more forceful. You can achieve this by sucking harder or by increasing the flicking movement of your tongue.*

As she reaches orgasm thrust your fingers into her vagina. (The erotic sages suggest thrusting a finger of the other hand into her anus, but this is a matter of personal taste and hygiene. Just make sure your finger is properly lubricated.)

The beginning of a relationship can be the most exciting time a couple ever spends with each other. Just make sure that you are forming good habits instead of ones that you will have to undo later. Hopefully, by following the suggestions and exercises in this chapter, you will ensure that the excitement and passion you feel now will continue for many, many years.

A man should kiss his wife's navel every day.

— Nell Kimball

Practice the discipline of delight—

Let no day go by without adding something

to the music of your experience.

— Sam Keen

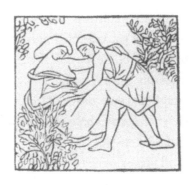

CHAPTER EIGHT

Summer Love:
Staying Sensual
and Integrating Passion
and the Family

☙

I deally, the "summer" phase of a relationship is a time when a couple settles into their life together. The newness of the relationship has worn off, but in its place partners find an easy comfort with each other. They are not as self-conscious around one another and they don't have to try as hard to impress each other. Life is good. The initial struggles of coming together as a couple are over. Partners have learned how to please each other sexually, and their love has grown to be as easy and comfortable as a summer day.

Unfortunately, once the excitement of the honeymoon period is over, many couples fall into habitual patterns of relating sensually and sexually. These can signal the beginning of the end of an exciting love life. Because they are no longer discovering and exploring, many couples find that their sex life becomes predictable and even boring. Moreover, the summer phase of a relationship is often when couples have children, which frequently puts a damper on their sexual relationship.

In this chapter you will find exercises designed to reignite your passions and restimulate your curiosity about each other's bodies as well as ways to help you integrate passion and family.

⑥ Sex and Bonding ⓔ

For your relationship to remain vital and fulfilling, you must maintain an intimate connection. According to Daniel Beaver, the author of *More Than Just Sex: A Committed Couples Guide to Keeping Relationships Lively, Intimate and Gratifying*, there are three ways in which this bonding normally occurs: through intimate verbal communication, touching, and sexual relations. [8]

Intimate Verbal Communication

This type of communication includes talking quietly together about how each of you is feeling, expressing your love and appreciation for each other, or teasing each other by talking explicitly about what you'd like to do with each other sexually.

Unfortunately, when time is limited, as it so often is for couples with children and/or busy careers, this form of bonding seldom occurs. And since many people feel embarrassed talking openly about their sexual feelings and desires, couples often have difficulty connecting in this way.

Touching

In the beginning of a relationship a lot of holding, touching, and kissing takes place between partners. In fact, some couples just can't seem to stop touching each other. Unfortunately, as time goes by couples seldom continue this behavior. Typically, the longer partners have been together, the less physical affection they exchange. This holding back is a result of many factors, a major one being our goal-oriented attitude that touching must automatically lead to intercourse. As the novelty wears off, when sex doesn't occur as spontaneously or as frequently, the amount of physical affection expressed by couples also diminishes.

Summertime couples tend to spend more time doing chores together than playing like they did when they were first together. When they do make time for sexual play, they tend to go straight for intercourse, because time is limited and they are tired from the day.

Sexual Relations

The third way a couple bonds is, of course, through sexual relations, primarily intercourse. Unfortunately, since most couples feel they don't have enough time to communicate verbally and since they have begun to restrict their expressions of affection, sexual intercourse often becomes the primary way in which they express their love for each other.

When this happens, a couple places too much weight on the sex act. Thus, what should be fun, relaxing, and enjoyable is turned instead into a proving ground for their love for each other. This type of pressure often causes the sexual relationship itself to deteriorate.

What happens when partners stop talking intimately, stop being affectionate, and eventually stop being sexual with each other? They become roommates. Their relationship withers. Whether or not the partners still get along, they cease to be a couple. Instead, they are two individuals living together, perhaps raising children together, but no longer feeling emotionally bonded. How long a relationship can last without bonding in love depends on the couple, but one thing is certain: without this type of bonding, the relationship eventually deadens, and reviving the old feelings becomes impossible. Daily maintenance of a love relationship is necessary to keep it vital and alive.

☾ A Caress a Day Keeps the Divorce Attorney Away ☽

While you may feel too tired at the end of the day to make love, make a commitment to spend a few minutes holding each other and sharing your feelings, making sure you share at least one thing you appreciate about each other. Share a sensuous bath or shower together. Spend a few minutes gently caressing each other. If you're too tired to make love, remind each other about a particularly exciting lovemaking experience you shared. Tease each other by describing what you'd like to do to each other and/or make plans for your next sexual escapade.

Remember that touching does not always have to be sexual. Through physical expressions of affection, such as hugging, holding hands, or caressing, you can express how you feel about each other any time. Couples who remain emotionally and physically close are often openly affectionate with each other. This affection serves to "prime the pump," so to speak, keeping the love and sexual energy between them alive.

Keeping sex strictly goal-oriented can have a negative impact on its frequency. After working all day trying to produce, perform, and achieve, the last thing you want to do is to continue working when you are finally home. This is why so many partners say, "I'm too tired tonight, honey," but stay up watching television or reading a book instead.

Being relaxed is the key to sexual pleasure. Sex is most rewarding when there is no pressure to perform, when we are simply being open to receiving and giving sexual pleasure. Then, instead of sex being an energy-draining experience, it becomes a way to reenergize our love relationship and ourselves. Unfortunately, many of us have difficulty allowing ourselves to have pleasure, since pleasure can often evoke guilt. Men especially often feel they should be producing, achieving, or making something happen. It's not okay to just experience pleasure unless they have done something to earn it.

Women who stay home with their infants or toddlers often complain about how tired they are from giving all day, as do women who work all day and then attend to their children and husbands in the evenings and on weekends. When a woman in this situation goes to bed at night and her husband initiates sexual activity, she may decline, saying she is too tired. But the truth may be that she sees sexual activity as a continuation of her day—more work and more giving of her energy. Unfortunately, by saying no to her husband, she is also saying no to herself. She is cutting off one of the few, and probably the best, opportunities to take care of herself emotionally and physically and one of her primary opportunities to experience pleasure.

To shift from a performance orientation to a pleasure orientation, try taking turns pleasuring each other. If one of you feels like having sex but the other feels too tired, agree that whoever is tired gets to play the role of the receiver. This means that instead of seeing sex with her husband as a time when she has to give some more, a wife can view lovemaking as an opportunity to receive sexual pleasure in whatever form she prefers. And instead of a man feeling like he is being called upon to perform one more task, a tired husband can simply lie back and be given to.

Once his or her batteries have been recharged, the tired spouse will often want to give pleasure back—but this should never be expected. Instead, pleasuring should be viewed as a nurturing experience only and as a way to maintain the emotional bond between you.

⑥ Make a Commitment ⑥

Unless you and your partner make a commitment to maintain your sensual and sexual relationship, you, like so many others, will discover that the sexual side of your relationship has withered and died like a neglected garden. Sit down and talk about how each of you feels about maintaining your sensual and sexual relationship. For example, on a scale of one to ten, how important is it for you to maintain a sexual relationship with your partner? Ask your partner the same question, and share your answers.

If it turns out that you agree on the importance of maintaining a sexual relationship, you are in luck. It should be fairly easy for you to remedy the situation by making a commitment and doing some planning.

However, it may turn out that your numbers are quite far apart and that one of you feels much stronger about the importance of sex in your relationship. If this is the case, you will need to continue talking and to be open to compromise. While it is normal for one partner to be more sexual than another, we all want and need physical and emotional connectedness. We all want to know we are loved. Connecting with each other on a sensual level isn't a luxury, it's a necessity if your relationship is to remain vital and intimate.

Even though one of you may not feel particularly sexual at a given time, connecting sensually may arouse sexual feelings. And even if it doesn't, you have made an important connection, one that will increase your level of emotional intimacy.

The following suggestions will help you maintain a sensually vital relationship, a relationship in which your emotional connection remains strong and is conducive to continued sexual sharing, exploration, and intimacy.

Make an agreement to share some kind of sensual experience at least once a week, whether or not you feel like having sex. This experience can be sharing a sensual shower or bath together, giving each other a sensual caress, or lying together and practicing synchronized breathing. Sharing any of these experiences will guarantee that you remain emotionally and sensually connected and will encourage sexual feelings to blossom, no matter how tired or stressed you feel.

You must remember to keep the pressure to perform off, however. Don't caress your partner only to turn her on. She will feel the pressure and will likely feel turned off and resentful, which might lead her to resist any future attempts at connecting. Remember that sexual feelings will arise only when you and your partner are feeling relaxed, trusting, and reconnected. Making a sensual connection with each other regularly will ensure this connectedness and trust and will create the space for sexual feelings to emerge.

Maintain your sensual refuge. In the beginning of this book, I discussed the importance of creating a room that is sensually stimulating and conducive to lovemaking. I can't stress enough the importance of creating this space together. To encourage and maintain a vital and exciting sexual relationship, you should decorate your bedroom in a way that invites intimacy and romance. Unfortunately, as a couple relaxes into a comfortable living situation, they often allow their sensual refuge to change into an office, dining room, or living room. Be sure not to do office work in your bedroom, thereby taking away from its romantic energy and infusing it with work energy instead. Likewise, it's best not to bring meals to bed or to eat snacks there in front of the television.

Take a look around your bedroom. Has it become cluttered and full of uninviting objects such as exercise machines and computers? The condition of your bedroom may reflect the condition of your love life. Brighten both up by clearing out unnecessary clutter so your love can shine through.

Do the colors in your bedroom soothe or excite you? Is your bed welcoming? Is your once-colorful bedspread fading? When was the last time you bought new sheets? Buying a new bedspread and sheets can enhance your sensual pleasure and represent a commitment to making lovemaking a priority in your life. The right artwork can help you to create a romantic or erotic mood, and strategically placed mirrors can give you a whole new perspective on your lovemaking. Make a project out of redecorating your bedroom to make it as sensually inviting and erotically exciting as possible.

Take a look at your bathroom as well. You can't expect to enjoy a sensual shower or bath together in a cluttered bathroom. Turn your bathroom into your own private spa with lots of thick towels, essential oils, and soft lighting. Bring a tape recorder or CD player into the bathroom with you and play your favorite music as you share a bath or shower, or place candles all around the tub as you soak together after a hard day's work.

Continue to experiment with various touches and to explore each other's bodies. The following suggestions and exercises will encourage you to once again view your partner's body as you did in the beginning of your relationship when you were so fascinated with and couldn't get enough of each other.

E x e r c i s e | The Epicurean Bath

You will want to save this very special bath for when you want to pamper your partner, communicate your deep love, or let her know how special she is.

Preparation: For the bath, you'll need candles, music, soft, luxurious towels, and liquid soap. For your love tray, you'll need champagne or sparkling water, champagne glasses, an ice bucket, a variety of exotic fruit (for example, figs, kiwi, mango, papaya, seedless grapes, strawberries, and cherries).

Begin by creating a romantic environment with candles and soft music. Run the bathtub for your lover, adding bubble bath or scent.

While the tub is filling, prepare the fruit and arrange them beautifully on the tray, then open the champagne and put it on ice.

When the bath is ready, call your lover in and help her into the bath, making a pillow with a rolled-up towel to go under her head. While she is enjoying the warmth of the water, retrieve your love tray from the kitchen and bring it in to her—naked.

Presenting her with the love tray, kneel beside her and ask if everything meets with her approval. When she says yes, open the champagne, pour it in the glasses, and make a toast along the lines of, "To the most beautiful woman in the world."

Still kneeling beside the tub, begin to feed your lover slices of fresh mango and papaya, smoothing some of the fruit gently but seductively across her lips and cheeks, down her neck and onto her chest, making sure to lick off the excess juices.

Teasingly dangle clusters of cherries and grapes over her head and slowly, slowly come close enough to her lips for her to reach them. Feed her strawberries and kiwi directly from your lips.

Sip some champagne and give your lover a champagne kiss, allowing the nectar to flow from your lips to hers. Take another sip and squirt champagne onto her neck, chest, and nipples.

For the grand finale, invite your lover to stand, step into the tub with her, and pour champagne between her breasts and your chest (or vice versa), allowing the cold, sparkling nectar to slither down your abdomens and genitals.

E x e r c i s e | **An Erotic Massage**

This sensual massage will cover the usual "hot spots," and also include many areas of the body that are not normally considered erogenous zones. Remember that all skin is erotic, and that wherever there are nerve receptors there is potential erotic sensation.

Preparation: Have your basic massage or caress supplies, such as oil and towels, on hand. Make sure the room is warm and that you will not be disturbed.

Remember to keep your touch light, much lighter than for a typical massage, and to make your movements very slow and sensuous. Refer to chapter 5 for a reminder of how to perform the caress technique.

After you have caressed a particular area, try breathing on that area and then titillating it with your tongue.

Try this sequence for maximum pleasure.

* *It's always a good idea to start with the back, since it is a neutral area and is guaranteed to relax your partner. Remember to use your palm, wrist, forearms, and the flats of your fingers. Warm the base of the spine by caressing in a circular motion. The nape of the neck is an erotic zone, especially for women, so experiment with kissing, licking, and blowing on this area.*

* *Make sure your partner's legs are comfortably wide apart, and slowly move up his legs and the insides of his thighs using the palms of your hands.*

* *Now move to the buttocks and make gentle, circular motions using your palms, wrists, and forearms. Move gently around and between the buttocks and on up to the waist using long strokes. Now is a good time to come close and breath on the area and tease it a bit with your tongue.*

* *Turn your partner over. Start by gently massaging his scalp and move down to stroke his forehead, jawline, and cheeks. Brush his eyelids with your tongue and lick the area between his eyebrows. Lightly brush the tips of your fingers over his lips. After you have gently massaged his earlobes, breathe close to his ear. Begin to lick, nibble, and suck his earlobes. Finally, let your tongue enter his ear.*

* *Move down to his chest and stomach. After caressing his chest, stimulate his nipples first by breathing on them and then by licking and nibbling. Tender tugging is usually pleasurable, as is caressing the nipple with the thumb as you hold it between the first two fingers. Move down to his stomach and caress it, using a clockwise circular motion. Circle around the navel with the flat of your palm and then put your tongue inside, moving your tongue in small circles.*

❖ *Move to his arms and hands. After making long strokes, press your middle finger into each palm and rotate it in circles. Suck and lick the outer edge of the little finger.*

❖ *Finally, move to his legs and feet. Use long, sweeping motions to caress his entire leg. Come in close as you caress his feet, and let your partner feel your breath. Suck and lick each of your partner's toes, finishing up by sucking on each of his big toes.*

❖ *Now bring your hot breath up to his genitals. Your partner will be melting with desire and eager to make love.*

Exercise | **More Erotic Experiences to Share**

If you feel you don't have the time or energy to give an erotic massage, then try these fun experiences.

❖ *Share a sensuous dinner at home (bring in take-out food from a local gourmet restaurant so that no one has to cook). Refer back to the instructions for a Sensuous Fruit Fest on page 63. Or make love using only your eyes as you sit across the table from each other. Tease each other as you sensuously eat your food. Lick your spoon seductively, dip your finger into your food and suck on it, and lick your lips invitingly. After dinner, take turns stripping for each other. Play music and include a striptease. Prolong actually having sex until you can't stand it any longer.*

❖ *On another occasion, allow your partner to slowly undress you, teasing you as he goes along.*

❖ *Slather oil, lotion, Jell-O, pudding, or whipped cream all over your own and your partner's body, and do a mutual massage using your entire bodies.*

⑥ How to Be a Parent and a Lover Too ⑨

Many couples who are contemplating parenthood fear that their sexual relationship will suffer if they have children, and for good reason. Couples who have children often have difficulty finding time for sex and are often so tired that they don't feel very sexual. It is also a fact that many women experience a lack of interest in sex after having a baby. Women generally need to take time for themselves after giving birth, to regain their sense of self until they will feel like a woman again, not just a mother. Because they are giving all their time to their new baby, sex may feel like just another act of giving. Moreover, the hormonal changes that occur up to a year after giving birth can decrease a woman's sex drive.

Men also sometimes experience a lessening of sexual drive following the birth of a child. Just as a new mother has to adjust to the newborn infant, men have to adjust to viewing their partner not only as a lover but also as a mother. Some men have expressed difficulty after watching the

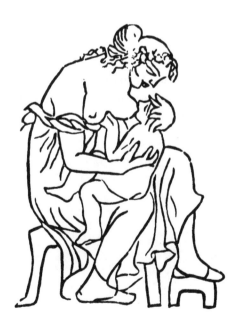

baby come out of their wife's vagina. One client told me, "I always associated that area of my wife's body with sex and arousal. Suddenly I now have another association with it and it seems to be getting in the way of my getting turned on." Still others refrain from approaching their wives out of concern about hurting them, and want to make certain they have fully recovered before attempting to resume active sexual relations.

For these reasons, couples who decide to become parents need sensuality more than ever if they want to remain sexual. Couples often need sensual "reminders" in order to get their juices flowing again. For example, Julia and Thomas, the parents of three small children, came into therapy complaining about no longer having the time or inclination for sex. I suggested several exercises, including the Sensuous Orange exercise from part 2.

They both really got into this particular exercise and ended up having a great time together both sensually and sexually. I suggested that they make oranges their private little secret, using an orange to sexually tease or flirt with each other or as a signal when they were feeling sexual.

This suggestion worked fabulously. Julia told me, "The orange has become our private message system. We can be having a typically noisy dinner with the kids and afterward one of us will pick out an orange from the fruit bowl and start slowly and seductively peeling it. No matter how harried or tired we're feeling we always have to laugh. And that simple gesture evokes so many positive memories for me that I can't help getting turned on most of the time."

E x e r c i s e | **Everyday Foreplay**

By incorporating a bit of foreplay into your everyday tasks and interactions, you will increase the possibility of feeling sexual with each other by the end of the day, no matter how tired you are. Here are just a few ideas.

❖ *Turn a simple "hello" into foreplay by talking to your partner in a low-pitched, seductive voice.*

❖ *Turn a simple hello kiss into foreplay with the deft use of your tongue.*

❖ *Whisper "I want you" as you brush by each other going through your daily routines.*

❖ *Seductively suck your finger as you make eye contact across a crowded room.*

❖ *Tell your partner when he looks especially sexy to you, whether he is just getting out of the shower or returning from the gym all sweaty.*

❖ *Help your partner undress as she changes out of her business clothes.*

❖ *Brush or comb your partner's hair.*

Making Sensuality a Priority

Just because you are a parent doesn't mean you don't need nurturing. In fact, you probably need it more than ever. And while it is natural for your sexuality to ebb and flow as you go through the various stages of parenthood, you will continue to be a sexual being with sexual needs.

Although it is difficult to maintain your sensual refuge when you have children, it is possible. No matter how crowded it gets as more and more kids come along, never allow your bedroom to become a nursery, a dining room, or a family room. Your bedroom should be your private sanctuary, a place you and your partner can go to reconnect, to comfort each other, and to make love. Therefore, for all intents and purposes, your bedroom should be off-limits to your children. You can't expect your sexual relationship to flourish when there are kids in bed with you watching television, eating ice cream, or doing their homework. All these activities should be confined to the living room, dining room, or family room.

This doesn't mean that you shouldn't allow your children to come into your room if they wake up frightened in the middle of the night or if they need extra comforting. But with the aid of a lock on the bedroom door or a rule about knocking before they enter, children should learn early on that their parent's bedroom is their private room where they shouldn't be disturbed. This may sound harsh, but if you are really serious about maintaining a healthy and exciting sexual relationship, these precautions are absolutely necessary. A fringe benefit is that your children will learn an important lesson about privacy and boundaries. Research shows that children who learn these lessons early in life actually fare better than children who do not. They grow up respecting the boundaries of others and insisting on their own boundaries being respected.

Summer love doesn't have to mean that you take a vacation from sex. As I have stressed throughout this book, to fully enjoy sex we must be relaxed, and it is in the summer that we tend to be the most laid back. Some of the most passionate sex can occur during the summer when the temperature soars and the days are long. Your love has grown deeper with time and with this deepening can come more passion and excitement—if you are willing to continue exploring, and if you make a commitment to continue having exciting sex throughout your relationship.

Love is like a violin. The music may stop

now and then, but the strings remain forever.

— JUNE MASTERS BACHER

Your body is the harp of your soul,

and it is yours to bring forth sweet music.

— KAHLIL GIBRAN

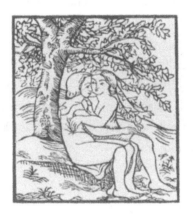

The Autumn
of Your Love:
The Joys of Midlife Sex

Autumn is a wonderful time of year. The air is cool and crisp, leaves turn brilliant shades of red, yellow, and orange. The crops have ripened and have been harvested, and the short, cold days of winter are still ahead. It is a time for celebration and relaxation.

The autumnal phase of a relationship can also be a wonderful time for a couple. Just as we traditionally celebrate the blessings of the harvest in autumn, it is a time when a couple can celebrate the harvest of their relationship—the intense closeness that comes only from loving and knowing each other intimately for many years.

If you have been diligent in your attempts at keeping your passion alive and at staying emotionally connected, as discussed in the last chapter, you have many years of fulfilling lovemaking ahead of you. You are still young enough—and probably healthy enough—to enjoy yourselves for many years. Even if you haven't been very diligent, this chapter offers ways to improve autumnal relationships.

Midlife: A Time of Transition

Just as autumn is a time of transition, preparing us for the shorter and cooler days of winter, midlife prepares us for the winter of our years. Just as we must say good-bye to the long, hot days of summer, so must we come to terms with our fading youth.

Midlife is a time of reevaluation and reassessment, both for individuals and for couples. It is during this time, when our children are grown and our careers established, that the all-important question, "What am I going to do with the rest of my life?" comes up. Some feel free to pursue interests that have been put aside for years, while others feel empty and lost.

As we reach midlife our priorities often shift. Faced with the reality of our aging bodies and our mortality, we often experience in midlife an emotional crisis that causes us to question our values, our belief systems, our accomplishments, and our lifestyles. Midlife is also a time when we take a closer look at our relationships and ask ourselves if we truly feel fulfilled—emotionally and sexually.

Couples who have been together for many years often need to get to know each other all over again. The same is true of couples who are reaching middle age, no matter how long they have been together. Along with the dramatic changes that can occur in our outlook on life, midlife can bring significant changes in our sexual desires and interests.

People in long-term relationships often make assumptions about each other based on what was true at the beginning of their relationship. Since sexual preferences can change, it is important to regularly check out these assumptions. For example, many people become less sexually inhibited in their middle years but fail to communicate this to their partners, as was the case with Donna and Brian.

Donna and Brian originally came to see me because Brian was going through what he called a "midlife crisis." He had grown severely depressed and complained that his life was meaningless and that his marriage was stagnant. He felt that Donna didn't really love him and that she only stayed with him because he was a good provider and because she was afraid to be alone.

Eventually, he got around to talking about sex. "We've been married for almost twenty years now and frankly, the passion has gone out of our sex life. I'd like to spice things up a bit with things like oral sex, but Donna's always tended to be a bit prudish, so I've just given up trying."

Much to Brian's surprise, Donna responded by saying, "My gosh, you're talking about how I was over ten years ago. I've changed a lot in the past ten years. I feel differently about it now."

"You mean you'd like to try it?" Brian asked tentatively.

"Yes, I actually would," Donna responded.

I am not saying that all Brian's problems were resolved because he and his wife were finally able to have oral sex. My point is that like so many other couples, they had failed to check in with each other about their current sexual likes and dislikes and had failed to communicate their current sexual needs. Without continuing, intimate communication you will not know your partner's changing needs, attitudes, and feelings, which can result in routine, predictable sex.

In this chapter I offer ways for midlife couples to check in with each other and to reassess their sexual and sensual relationship. This process will include getting to know each other's bodies all over again, taking into consideration that important changes have occurred with aging, and communicating about what kind of sexual relationship you would like.

We all know that some men react to midlife by desperately trying to recapture their youth, including having sexual affairs with younger women. While this situation is obviously upsetting to these men's wives, it can be equally upsetting to the husbands, who value their marriage but feel stirrings that seem to be beyond their control. This phenomenon also occurs among women, but to a lesser degree. This is true for several reasons. Until relatively recently, it was socially unacceptable for an older woman to become involved with a younger man, and even today it is less acceptable than the other way around. Also, in the past most women didn't take care of themselves the way many do today and consequently weren't as attractive to younger men. This, coupled with the fact that most midlife women don't have the money and power that midlife men have, is why fewer young men would be interested in older women. It is vital that couples confront this possibility head-on, by openly discussing their fears and by tackling the core causes of the problem together.

Another aspect of midlife may threaten even the closest of relationships: both men and women can change radically in how they view their sexual relationship and in how they function sexually. Whereas the typical woman may have focused primarily in the past on the emotions surrounding sex, she may now begin to focus on and develop the physical aspects of her sexuality. She may no longer need to be "in the mood" or to need sweet talk, flowers, or romance to arouse her interest. On the other hand, a man who was once preoccupied with his physical needs may now find that the emotional aspects of sexuality have become far more important to him. His sexual response may now come only when physical and emotional conditions are just right. In this sense, many women and men actually exchange roles.

A woman's sexual potential during midlife is limitless. She can make love for hours, enjoy sexual activities she may not have considered before, and experience spectacular orgasms, including multiple orgasms and orgasms brought on by the stimulation of her G-spot. Her sexual blossoming may in turn threaten her mate, who may feel his own sexual power is declining. Men often act out this fear by rejecting women their own age for a younger woman whom they feel will be less demanding.

A man needs to be reassured that you find him just as desirable when he has a "soft-on" as when he has a hard-on and that you appreciate his increased skill at ejaculatory control. Tell him that you love the increased emotionality that comes more easily to him now, and allow him to be passive at times by taking a more active role in lovemaking yourself.

A woman needs to be assured that it's fine for her to violate the rules of female passivity that she has been taught, that you appreciate her taking the initiative at times, and that you still find her attractive, even with her aging skin or Cesarean scars.

For a midlife relationship to survive, both partners must agree to openly discuss their feelings, including their hopes, fears, and desires concerning the emotional and sexual side of their relationship. The following suggestions and exercises will help set the stage for such sharing.

Exercise | **The Sex Talk**

Set aside a time and a place to discuss your sexual relationship. Choose a setting that is conducive to such a discussion. You may want to begin the conversation at a favorite restaurant where you both feel comfortable, or during a long walk or drive. Just make sure you won't be distracted or interrupted and that one or both of you is not preoccupied with something else.

You may wish to use this book to initiate the discussion. Or you might prefer to make a special appointment to talk. Make sure you don't bring up the subject during an argument or disagreement or after a frustrating day. Picking a time when you and your partner are both relaxed and when you feel close to each other will enhance the possibility of good communication.

You can make it easier on both of you by first reassuring your partner that you want to continue the relationship or by expressing your love. You may want to say that you don't believe you have adequately communicated your needs in the past or reassure your partner that you are not blaming her or him. Then begin to discuss your concerns about your sexual relationship, any needs that are not being met, and the changes you wish to see. Finally, encourage your partner to share any suggestions that might make lovemaking more satisfying for both of you.

Your talk should include issues such as:

❖ *How important is a good sexual relationship at this point in your life?*

❖ *What do you desire from a sexual relationship?*

❖ *How have you changed regarding your sexual desires or attitudes?*

❖ *What do you feel is missing from your sexual relationship?*

❖ *What have you always wanted to do sexually that you have never done? Do you consider this a fantasy only or is it something you would like to pursue?*

It is very important that you talk openly, and equally important that you really listen to each other. Interestingly, people who have had extramarital affairs often say that they did so as much because someone else took an interest in what they had to say as they did to have sex with someone other than their spouse.

E x e r c i s e | **Asking for What You Want**

Sadly, many people reach the autumnal phase of their relationship without having ever told their partner exactly what pleases them sexually. If this is the case with you, ask yourself, "What do I have to lose at this point? At my age, isn't it high time for me to finally get what I want?"

The following exercise will help you get past any resistance you may have to asking for exactly what you want. It will also help you learn to give clear, specific directions on how you like to be touched.

1. Begin by giving your partner explicit instructions on how to massage what is usually considered a nonsexual part of your body such as your back, shoulders, arms, hands, or feet. For example, you might say, "I'd like you to rub my back and shoulders. I can take quite a lot of pressure, so you don't have to be gentle. Spend a little more time with my right shoulder because it's particularly sore."

2. As your partner massages you, continue giving instructions and feedback. Don't worry about hurting your partner's feelings and don't feel you should just be grateful for your partner's efforts. You deserve to be touched in exactly the ways you prefer. Don't stop instructing until he gets it just right. Your instructions and feedback may go something like this: "Could you rub a little harder? Yes, that feels good. Ahhh, that's great. Now move a little to the left. A little further. Now you've got it. Ouch! Yes, that hurts but it feels good. Lighten up just a little. Oh yeah. That's great."

3. Switch roles so that your partner can practice asking for what he wants.

4. Now it is your turn again, and this time you will be teaching your partner how to stimulate you sexually. Start by choosing an area of your body you would like to have stimulated such as your mouth, breasts, neck, ears, or genitals. Acting as if your partner has never stimulated this area before, give her detailed instructions on how to do it. The goal isn't to become sexually aroused but to give specific, clear instructions. If need be, supplement your words with hands-on instructions.

   Here's an example of a woman giving her partner instructions on how to pleasure her clitoris. "I'd like you to touch my clitoris. Make sure to use some lubricant. Start by gently touching my thighs and the outside of my vagina. That feels good. Now begin to gently caress my outside lips. Use plenty of oil. That's good. Just take your time. Now spread my lips apart and put some lubricant on my clitoris. Just stroke it gently. A little lighter. That's right. Just continue stroking it lightly like that. Now try using your thumb. Oh, that feels good. Press a little harder. That's perfect."

   Once your partner is thoroughly "trained," you can dispense with the instructions and concentrate on the pleasure. Keep in mind, however, that many people don't like the same touch all the time. They may prefer a lighter touch or a stronger one depending on their mood, their emotional state, or their physical condition. Some women, for example, may prefer a different touch depending on whether they are ovulating or experiencing PMS.

We would think that by this point in their lives, couples would have stopped putting pressure on themselves and/or their partners to perform a certain way or to have a particular type of orgasm. But ironically, it is often at midlife that couples focus on performance the most. For example, men who cannot achieve an erection as quickly as they once did often begin to feel an increased pressure to perform. Unless a woman is understanding and reassuring, she can add to the pressure. And men who once seemed to have all the patience in the world helping their lover achieve an orgasm may tire more easily and thus become impatient. This impatience in turn adds to the pressure a woman already feels to achieve an orgasm.

The genital caress exercise will serve to remind you both that sex is best enjoyed when the pressure is off. Please refer to page 156 for full instructions. During and after the genital caress are also good times to update each other about the types of touches you like and to ask your partner to touch you in a way that he or she may have neglected for some time.

E x e r c i s e | **Spreading the Pleasure**

Earlier in this book you learned a technique for spreading the pleasure. This exercise is a variation on that theme and is especially effective for midlife couples. This spreading technique will help to take the pressure to perform off each other and will allow you to feel ecstatic feelings that will bond you together emotionally.

You can do this spreading technique after completing the genital caress discussed on page 156–159 or as a variation of it.

❖ *Take the positions described on pages 157 with the passive partner lying facing the active partner, legs over legs.*

❖ *The active partner will begin by caressing his or her partner's outer thighs with long, slow, sensuous caressing strokes, using plenty of oil. Then move to the tops of the thighs, and only after a few minutes, to the inner thighs.*

When the male is the active partner:

❖ *Using lots of lubrication, slowly move your hand over your lover's pubic mound and gently move your fingers over her outer labia. After a few minutes, move to the inner lips, and continue to stroke with gentle, light movements. Now slowly move to her clitoris and lightly caress it, making sure your fingers are sufficiently lubricated.*

❖ *After spending a few minutes with her clitoris, move back out to the inner lips, then to the outer lips. Now brush over the mons and spread the pleasure up to her hips and stomach. Caress her stomach briefly and move up to her chest. Remember to use long, smooth, gentle strokes. Caress her chest up as far as you can reach and then begin to make your way down the body once again.*

❖ *When you have reached her genitals again, begin to caress the area where her pubic hair grows and brush over the entire area. Then once again, using plenty of lubricant, begin to caress the outer, then inner lips, and finally, the clitoris. Do this for a few minutes, noting your lover's arousal. When she seems to be reaching a more intense arousal, begin to caress her inner thighs once again, making sure you move all the way down to her knees. Finally, move to the top of her thighs and her outer thighs. Rest your hands there for a few moments before beginning the process all over again—thighs, mons, outer lips, inner lips, clitoris.*

❖ *Do this spreading technique at least two complete times before focusing all your attention on her genitals.*

When the female is the active partner:

❖ *Using plenty of lubrication, slowly begin caressing your lover's penis, making long strokes downward starting at the head of the penis and moving all the way down the shaft. After a few minutes, move to his scrotum and begin gently touching it with the tips of your fingers. You may also want to lift up the scrotum and gently caress the underside.*

❖ *Move back to the penis and once again begin caressing very, very slowly, using long strokes. No matter how aroused your partner becomes, do not speed up your strokes but continue at a relaxed pace. Remember that your purpose is to spread the pleasure, not to help him reach orgasm. If he ejaculates, simply wipe him off with a towel and move on to the next step.*

❖ *Now begin to spread the pleasure by moving to his hips and stomach. Caress his stomach and then move up to his chest, remembering to use long, smooth, gentle strokes. Caress his chest up as far as you can reach and then begin to make your way down the body once again.*

❖ *When you reach his genitals again, begin to caress the area where his pubic hair grows and gently brush over the entire area. Then, using lots of lubricant, begin to caress the scrotal area. Finally, return to the penis and caress with long, slow strokes. Do this for a few minutes or until your lover seems to be reaching a heightened state of arousal. Now begin caressing his inner thighs using long strokes moving all the way to his knees. Finally, move to the top of his thighs and outer thighs. Gently rest your hands there for a few moments before beginning the process all over again—thighs, scrotum, penis. . . .*

⑥ As Your Body Changes ⑥

Aging is accompanied by all types of changes in the body, including hormonal changes. We begin to sprout hair in odd places and our skin becomes drier and begins to wrinkle. With these changes often come insecurities and fears concerning our physical and sexual attractiveness.

Your body image has a tremendous impact on your ability to enjoy your sexual relationship. People who feel flawed on the outside often feel undesirable sexually. Signs of aging can have a tremendous effect on your sexual self-esteem unless you actively work toward alleviating feelings of embarrassment or self-hatred.

The following suggestions will facilitate a growing acceptance of your body and your natural bodily responses:

❖ *Look at yourself nude in a full-length mirror. Doing this will undoubtedly be difficult at first, perhaps because of embarrassment, self-criticism, or self-hatred, but continue to do it until you feel a little more comfortable. Then find at least one positive thing to say out loud to yourself regarding your body. For example, you might say, "My body is strong and healthy" or "My body is well proportioned."*

❖ *Find at least one part of your body that you like, and very lovingly apply lotion or oil to that part. Again, say at least one positive statement about that part of your body, such as "I have pretty hands" or "My legs are strong."*

❖ *Make a habit of spending a few minutes every day caressing your skin and rubbing lotion on yourself. Give yourself positive affirmations as you do so, such as "My body is strong and healthy. I deserve to feel all kinds of wonderful bodily sensations."*

You should do all these exercises when you are alone. You may feel uncomfortable, so move through them at your own pace, since it is important that you feel in control of the experience. The more you do them, the more comfortable you will feel.

Your body image will not change overnight, but in repeating these exercises you will notice a change, and this will give you the encouragement you need to explore still further, possibly with your partner.

Women in particular have a difficult time with aging because of the negative cultural messages that abound concerning women and aging. Thus, you may continually need to work toward greater body acceptance by looking in the mirror, focusing on positive aspects of your appearance, and then complimenting yourself out loud. But you also need your partner's love and support to overcome the many negative and false assumption that surround us, chiefly that women with wrinkles, extra pounds on their hips, or gray hair are past their sexual prime. If your mate internalizes and expresses our culture's ageism, he will only become part of the problem instead of part of the solution.

Exercise | **Improving Your Body Image**

Although most men don't worry as much as women about the effects of aging on their physical appearance, they tend to have fears about declining sexual performance. Many men feel undesirable if they can't get erections when they want them and view this inability as a sign of weakness.

Make it safe to talk to each other about your fears concerning aging. When you both feel rested and open to each other, share the following information:

❖ *What do you most fear about aging?*

❖ *How do you feel aging has affected or will affect our sexual relationship?*

❖ *How do you feel about your body? Do you still feel physically and sexually attractive?*

Your Favorite Things

Many middle-aged people prefer to have sex in the dark out of embarrassment or out of fear that their partner will catalogue their physical faults even as they are making love. But according to several studies—as well as my own experience as a clinician—most people are surprised to discover that their partners are far less critical of their body than they are themselves. When we are critical of a certain part of our bodies, we tend to assume that everyone else is as well. But in reality, the parts of our bodies that embarrass us—a scar, sagging breasts, a large butt—are frequently endearing to our partners.

The following exercises will serve to assure you that no matter what shape you are in or how old you are, there are parts of your body that your partner still adores.

Exercise | **Your Favorite Body Parts**

When we are lovingly touching our partner, we tend to get caught up in the sensations and emotions, not on how our partner looks. But most of us forget this. Because so many of us are self-conscious about our body as we age, we focus only on how our body looks to our partner instead of how it feels to our partner. This exercise will remind you that sex involves more than visual stimulation.

1. Take turns giving each other a full-body caress, using your favorite massage and/or essential oils.

2. Once you have completed the body caress, go back to the area of your partner's body that you enjoyed touching the most. Continue caressing this area for as long as you like. Sink into the pleasure.

3. As you continue to touch this area, begin to share with your partner why you like it so much and how it makes you feel when you touch it.

4. Ask your partner how it feels to receive your touch and to witness your enjoyment.

Exercise | **Show and Tell and Smell**

In addition to being self-conscious about how their body looks as they grow older, many people worry about their body odor being offensive to their partner. This exercise will remind you that when someone loves you, they also love your smell. And it will also help you feel more comfortable undressing in front of each other.

1. You will begin this exercise by allowing your partner to undress you. While you may feel self-conscious at first, try to get into it, making it as titillating as possible. After your partner has undressed you, it is your turn to do the same. Once again, really get into it, making it a sensual experience.

2. Now lie down facing each other, completely nude. Take turns sharing what part of each other's body you like to look at the most. Say why you like to look at it, what it does to you, how it makes you feel. If looking at this particular part of the body turns you on, tell your partner this.

3. Finally, share with each other what parts of each other's body smells the best to you. You may find that though you have become more self-conscious of how your body smells, these very smells may be a turn-on for your partner, or they may just be a comforting reminder to them of you.

Most people are surprised to hear what their partner chooses as their favorite part of the body to touch, look at, or smell. Often these parts are the very ones they personally dislike the most. Rarely does one partner pick the part of the body that the other partner likes the most about themselves.

You Are So Beautiful

We all need to know that our partner still finds us physically attractive, no matter how old we get. The song *You Are So Beautiful,* originally sung by Joe Cocker, is many couples' favorite, because it so eloquently expresses their deep love for each other. The next time you are in a music store, buy the tape or CD of this song. Then pick a special time to play the song for your partner, a time when you know she or he is feeling especially unattractive or when you feel particularly loving. A variation on this theme is to repeat "you are so beautiful" to your partner as you make love.

⑥ Added Pleasures ⑨

Although I believe that intimacy and sensuality are the greatest aphrodisiacs, sometimes these elements can be enhanced in a relationship when we learn certain sexual techniques. The important thing is that your focus remains on communicating your love to each other and on connecting or reconnecting with all your senses—not on performance.

E x e r c i s e | **Pleasuring a Male Partner**

According to several surveys, fellatio is what men most often say is lacking in their sex lives. If you have never given oral sex to your mate, perhaps you should try. (You can refer to the instructions given in chapter 7.) In addition, try the following techniques to bring added pleasure and excitement to the experience.

❖ *Hold your partner's penis in your hand as if you were holding a flute. Imagine that you are playing a song with your fingertips. Now roll your fingers at the base in a rhythm from index finger to little finger.*

❖ *Play "guess the caress" using different stimuli (feather, silk, fur, oil) while he, with his eyes closed, tries to guess what you are doing. A variation is to use various edible lubricants such as chocolate, honey, or peanut butter and have him guess what you are using. If you feel so inclined, you may want to try a taste test yourself.*

❖ *Women aren't alone in liking vibrators. Try using one behind his scrotum on the perineum.*

Exercise | **Pleasuring a Female Partner**

Men often tend to be goal oriented, and touch their partner's breasts or genitals just to get her aroused or to get her to perform a certain sexual act. But women often want to be touched for touch's sake, with no pressure. As my client Laurie told me, "Men are always in such a hurry to go further. Before we were married, Ted always pressured me to have intercourse. Then once we got married he was always rushing to have sex so he could have an orgasm and go to sleep. Now that he's older he's always in a rush because he's afraid he'll lose his erection."

As many women know, patience makes a great lover. A touch that aims to get a woman to feel what her partner wants her to feel is much less pleasurable than a touch that gently stimulates her whole body before focusing on her breasts or vulva, a touch that gently invites her to go just a step further.

In therapy, Ted learned to pay attention to Laurie's cues and to let her wait just a little longer for each touch. Rather than zeroing in on her breasts or genitals when he felt like making love, he learned to tease her and wait a little, and then to wait a little longer. When he finally did touch her genitals, she was more than ready. The following exercise will teach you another teasing—and pleasing—technique.

❖ *Usually when a woman says she wants you inside her, you feel she is ready for you. But don't be too quick to satisfy her desire. The longer you wait, the more pleasure she will get once you do enter her. According to tantric teachings, it's best to wait until her vagina is on fire with the desire to consume your penis.*

   The typical scenario might go like this. You've been stimulating her clitoris for a while. She is getting very excited. She may have already had an orgasm. She whispers to you, "I want you" or "come inside me." Instead of satisfying her desire immediately, wait. Continue stimulating her.

   Seconds later you may hear another whisper, louder this time. "What are you waiting for? I want you inside me."

Wait still longer until her tone changes and desire has taken her over completely. "Oh God, I want you! Now! Please!" She may start pushing your hand away from her clitoris or she may grab for your penis. Moaning with desire, she is now ready.

Of course, every woman is different. Some women are quieter than others, and you may have to read your lover's body language to tell when she is really ready.

⑥ Advanced Techniques for Experienced Lovers ⑥

They say that middle-aged women and men make the best lovers. They have years of experience behind them and they still have the good health and stamina to bring their lover to his or her knees. Here are some advanced techniques to add to your repertoire, techniques that are bound to thrill even the most jaded partner.

Advanced Techniques to Please Him

❖ *Pleasure your partner's prostate to provide a new and unique experience. The prostate is equivalent to the woman's G-spot. It can be stimulated indirectly by pressing on the prostate point in the middle of the perineum between the scrotum and the anus, or directly through the anus.*

Once your partner is aroused, press at different points near the middle of the area between the scrotum and anus and ask him how it feels. Press firmly with the tips of your fingers or thumb. (Your nails need to be short for this technique.) If you find that a certain spot feels especially good, make a mental note for the future. Also, try varying the pressure and ask him how each shift feels. When he is aroused you may be surprised at how hard you can push on this point.

If you are going to stimulate him through the anus, it is important that you use a latex surgical glove or finger. Use plenty of water-based lubricant, and go very slowly. It is not unreasonable to ask that your partner take a light enema just before you begin.

Stimulating the prostate gland can not only lead to an exceptional orgasm but it is also a reliable way to prolong erection and delay ejaculation. Rhythmic pressure on the prostate just before orgasm is reached can also help a man stay on the verge of an orgasm for many minutes. You can also stimulate the prostate point during your partner's orgasm to extend it. Finally, a rapid, rhythmic alternation of applying pressure to the prostate and penis can lead to a considerable prolongation of orgasm. Alternating in this way takes time and practice to develop and will also increase his sensitivity.

❖ *This technique is from the Kama Sutra, the famous ancient Indian erotic text. When you sense that your partner is approaching ejaculation, slap his buttocks and his chest with your open palm. If you slap with enough force, his ejaculation will be delayed (of course, do not slap him so hard that you injure him). Repeat the technique until he achieves orgasm.*

Advanced Techniques to Please Her

❖ *Discovering and stimulating your partner's sacred spot or G-spot can add both an exciting and a deeply satisfying element to her sexual experience. This part of the vagina is mentioned in the Kama Sutra; but Dr. Ernest Graffenberg, whom the G-spot is named after, first described it to the Western world more than thirty years ago.*

The woman should empty her bladder before beginning. It is believed that the optimal time to stimulate the sacred spot is after a woman has already orgasmed via her clitoris. This is not only because she will be more relaxed and open but because sacred-spot stimulation brings the deepest satisfaction when a woman is either fully aroused or has just had an orgasm.

To locate your lover's sacred spot, first introduce one or two fingers into her vagina, palm toward you, facing front. If she is not sufficiently lubricated, apply a lubricant to your finger and the first inch of her vagina. Curl your fingers so that the tips touch the upper ceiling of the vagina. Using a "come here" motion, slowly pull your fingers toward the front of the vagina. Her sacred spot will be located somewhere between her pubic bone and the front of the vaginal ceiling. It may feel a little rougher than the surrounding flesh.

If she suddenly feels an urge to urinate, you have probably found the right place. Continue to stroke with a soft, rhythmic motion. Steadily move your index and middle fingers up and back as well in and out. Usually, after a few minutes, her urge to urinate will give way to great pleasure. She may feel like she has to urinate, but the only liquid to be released will be the kama salila, *or the "juice of love." Most women will need you to continue for at least five minutes or until she experiences the deeper, stronger sacred-spot orgasm.*

Some women find that being rhythmically stimulated back and forth between the clitoral bud and the sacred spot extends their orgasm, either in the form of a lasting plateau or as multiple orgasms. Experiment and encourage her to tell you what she likes. Some women don't want to be touched or stimulated further after a powerful orgasm.

Advanced Techniques for Both Sexes: Tantric Massage

According to tantric teachings, during tantric massage your hands connect with the physical, emotional, and spiritual levels of your beloved. It is believed that through this contact you can communicate directly with your lover's heart and soul.

❖ *Prepare a sacred space with candlelight and essential oils or incense (see chapter 6 for directions).*

❖ *Begin by touching your partner's face. Do so with reverence, for this is a very personal part of her body. Use light flowing strokes, circling over her cheeks and around her chin.*

❖ *Stroke her abdomen using circular strokes to relax emotional and physical tensions that can inhibit the flow of sexual energy. Approach this vulnerable area with care and allow your touch to deepen the trust between you.*

❖ *Stimulate the valley between her breasts, a frequently neglected erotic zone for both men and women. Caressing or rubbing this area is said to stimulate the thymus gland, which in turn opens the heart and enhances our ability to love others and ourselves.*

❖ *According to tantric teachings, a flexible spine enables sexual energy to rise during lovemaking. Help relax your partner's spine by gliding your hands down on either side of it several times. Use shorter and deeper movements with your thumbs to release tightness closer to the bone.*

❖ *Apply loving strokes on and around her genital area, communicating both respect and love. Your partner will feel the sincerity and warmth of your touch, which will create both trust and relaxation.*

⑤ Exciting Your Senses and Revitalizing Your Sexual Relationship ⑥

As we discussed in the first part of this book, an exciting, vital, fulfilling sex life requires you to be in touch with all your senses. Unfortunately, the repetition and familiarity of a long-term relationship can dull our senses. Therefore, in order to revitalize them, you may need to be more experimental than you were years ago. While kissing and fondling may have once been all that was necessary to excite you and your partner, you may now need to step outside your normal routine and introduce unusual or exotic practices or objects into your lovemaking. The following suggestions will stimulate your senses and jump-start your libido.

Sight

❖ *Maximize your sensual pleasure by looking deeply into your lover's eyes. Many partners in long-term relationships avoid each other's gazes or look at each other for only a few fleeting seconds. Risk intense intimacy with your partner by maintaining eye contact for a full sixty seconds the next time you make love.*

❖ *Consider watching erotic films together. While we have traditionally believed that men are more sexually aroused by visual stimulation than women, we are coming to realize more and more that women are also strongly affected by what they see. Though some women say they are aroused by hard-core pornography, according to at least one study, most women prefer to watch soft-core films (depicting sex within the context of a loving relationship) to hard-core films (depicting sex only, with no love or affection).*

Erotica can also be extremely stimulating but without the after-effects of shame, guilt, and self-loathing that many people, especially women, experience with pornography. I define erotica as "literary or artistic works having an erotic theme or quality." This is a very broad definition, but the major distinction between works of erotica and pornography is that erotica does not portray women in degrading or subservient ways, and the violence inherent in pornography is absent.

In recent years a few video companies, such as Femme Productions, have begun to produce erotic films that are less objectionable than the standard films of this type. Although they contain explicit sex scenes, these are not demeaning to women, the actors treat one another with respect, and the woman's pleasure is given as much importance as the man's. The company Good Vibrations also offers a service called the Sexuality Library, which includes mail-order videos, erotic literature, erotic art, and educational material (see Resources).

Sound

❖ *Share your feelings for each other using loving, romantic, and erotic words. Search for poetry and erotica that best expresses your feelings toward your partner and your most secret desires. Try reading erotic stories or poetry out loud to one another. Erotic poetry, in addition to igniting your passion, can connect you to your deepest feelings and teach you erotic truths. The book* Passionate Hearts: The Poetry of Sexual Love *is a personal favorite, since it celebrates healthy sexual intimacy. Edited by Wendy Maltz, a sex educator and therapist, it not only provides some beautiful poetry but also provides excellent models for healthy relating.*

❖ *For those so inclined, I recommend writing poetry and erotica of your own. Then read the words of love and lust that are in your heart out loud to each other.*

❖ *Tantalize each other with explicit descriptions of what you intend to do to each other. Even though you may prefer romantic conversations in bed to explicit sex talk, consider venturing out of your comfort zone and using the words and phrases that are most exciting to your partner. Although they may not initially be a turn-on for you, your partner's excitement may become contagious.*

Taste

❖ *Although using whipped cream and chocolate syrup has become a cliché, many couples swear by it. There are many other ways to titillate your sense of taste, by using various flavors such as peanut butter, honey, yogurt, butterscotch sauce, flavored oils, or edible lubricants.*

Smell

❖ Remembering that smell has the ability to elicit memories, use some familiar scents to stimulate your lovemaking, such as the perfume you wore when you first met, the scent from her favorite flowers, or fresh pine sprigs to remind you of your honeymoon in the mountains.

❖ Since our sense of smell can change over the years, embark on an adventure to a fragrance store or a store that sells essential oils and pick out scents that are stimulating to you both.

❖ Incorporate essential oils that are known to be aphrodisiacs into your lovemaking. These essential oils include anise, black pepper, bergamot, clary sage, fennel, frankincense, geranium, jasmine, ginger, juniper, lime, myrrh, orange, rose, patchouli, sandalwood, vetiver, and ylang-ylang. The best aphrodisiacs make use of the brain, since this is where the sexual center is located, as are memories and hormone regulatory functions. Aromatic baths, massage oils, and inhalation are recommended because they also encourage intimacy and touch. Essential oils can also be used in the Jacuzzi, bath, or shower, and sprinkling a few drops onto the bedsheets and using candles, diffusers, and room sprays are other ideas to experiment with.

❖ Experiment with various exotic smells by burning incense and scented candles.

Touch

❖ Take turns experimenting with different kinds of touches on various parts of your body until you come up with at least three especially thrilling "touch zones" and types of touch that you each prefer.

❖ Lick your partner's body all over. Experiment with love bites and nibbling and observe the reaction you get.

❖ Electrify your sense of touch by experimenting with various textures such as silk, satin, feathers, or temperatures such as warm towels or ice.

⑥ The Soul of Sex ◎

Although midlife can have its downside, it offers many positives as well. With midlife often come a mellowing and an appreciation for life that most younger people do not possess. You have grown to appreciate the finer things in life more, such as music, art, literature, and nature. Sharing these things can bring you together in ways that nothing else can, especially when they are combined with sensuality.

Using music, art, and nature as the catalyst, begin to open your souls to each other. Begin by discovering or rediscovering exactly what types of nature, music, art, or literature touch your soul.

❖ *Share the music, art, and literature that now hold particular meaning for you, and incorporate them into your lovemaking.*

❖ *Spend some time looking through old records or tapes for the music that was part of your youth or that reminds you of when you first met. Play the music together and reminisce about old times. Dance together the way you once did. Play the music while you caress each other and while you make love.*

❖ *Share your favorite classical music.*

❖ *Plan a night around listening to opera (if you both like it.) For example, cook an Italian meal together while listening to* La Traviata. *Sip wine together afterward and talk about how the music made you feel. Choose another opera to make love by.*

❖ *Write love letters to each other. Writing love letters is a time-honored way to express your most vulnerable feelings toward each other, feelings you may be unable to express any other way. It is a way to go on record with your love, to reinstate your commitment. These letters will in turn engender loving feelings in your partner.*

Finally, share with your partner the experiences in your life that were particularly meaningful to you and explain why these experiences held such intensity or depth. Promise each other to make an effort to reexperience some of these life experiences and to cultivate new, but similar, ones.

Don't let the loss of summer or your fears of winter prevent you from appreciating the joys of autumn. Celebrate your love, the obstacles you've overcome together, and the fact that you still have the time to explore new avenues of intimacy and sensuality.

Midlife can be an exciting time for couples who are open to change and to rediscovering each other. By following the suggestions in this chapter, you will infuse your relationship with new excitement and deepen your intimacy.

Contrary to public opinion, lovemaking is not enjoyed best by those who are young and physically beautiful but by those who are mature enough to love and accept themselves and their partners physically, emotionally, and spiritually. It's never too late to learn to love yourself and your partner more deeply. In fact, as we age our ability to love increases, so that at fifty we can love more deeply and fully than we could at the tender age of twenty.

Age does not protect you from love.

But love, to some extent, protects you from age.

— Jeanne Moreau

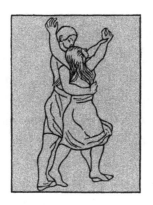

CHAPTER TEN

Winterlove:
Growing Older and
Growing Closer

Winter is a special time indeed. Even though winter brings with it shorter days and cooler temperatures, it is also a time when we tend to draw closer to our loved ones, when the home fires burn just a little bit brighter.

Winter love allows you to appreciate the good years you've had together, to reminisce about when you first met, and to evaluate the changes you've made in your relationship.

Older couples have special issues when it comes to their sensual and sexual relationship. On the upside, many have learned (often by necessity) to slow down and enjoy the sensual side of their relationship. On the down-side, our senses age with us and are not as keen as they once were, and we tend to experience more physical limitations. As a result, we may experi-ence a cooling of our sexual relationship.

In this chapter you will find suggestions and exercises specifically designed to help older couples refine and revitalize their senses and learn to appreciate the sensual pleasures of simple intimacy. To accommodate aging muscles and bones, I will suggest sensual experiences that are less physically demanding than some of those given earlier in this book. I also encourage older couples to take advantage of the fact that they have fewer demands on their time and energy and can therefore devote more time to each other, and I suggest ways for older lovers to express their deepest love for each other.

⑥ The Good News ◎

The good news is that we are coming to realize that getting older does not automatically mean an inevitable loss of sexual desire or desirability. Although we still struggle with stereotypes about aging, such as the idea that women over fifty are no longer sexy or that older men who can't "get it up" as readily as younger men have nothing to offer a woman sexually, more and more of us understand that as our bodies age, our hearts and our sexuality blossom in new ways. Many women don't come into their own sexually until they reach their fifties or sixties. Men who are no longer young often become more sensitive lovers because of their increased emotional openness. Many older women have reported feeling far deeper orgasms than they were ever able to in their youth and experiencing multiple orgasms for the first time. Many men love the fact that their erections last longer than when they were younger.

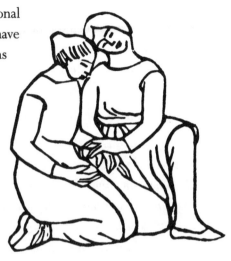

Another benefit of aging is that old fears about sex may dissipate or disappear altogether. A person who disliked oral sex because he or she was taught it was dirty or "unnatural" may now have enough distance from their childhood training to view it with a new openness. A man who was reluctant to become emotionally vulnerable when he was younger may now have the courage and maturity to do so. And a woman who may have felt pressured by her husband to experiment sexually earlier in their marriage may now feel secure and loved enough to risk it.

Like a fine wine, you have grown rich and ripe with your advancing years. You have learned that love takes time and so does good sex. One of the joys of being retired is that you no longer have to show up at the office at nine. You can stay up late at night making love, or you can make love first thing in the morning. You can take a nap together in the afternoon and then spend hours together touching and loving and experiencing "afternoon delights." You are in no hurry. You can take long, sensual baths, showers, and Jacuzzis together. You can take all day bringing each other to new heights of ecstasy.

⑥ Opportunities for Love ⑥

Though you may have been too busy making a living or raising a family to devote much time to each other, now you have all the time in the world to express how much you love and appreciate each other. Here are a few suggestions.

❖ *Give each other a leisurely shampoo.*

❖ *Float each other in the pool or Jacuzzi—a very special and loving activity. Ask your partner to float on her back in the water. You can help her stay afloat by holding her against your body and by holding her up with one hand under her neck and the other under her back. Slowly, gently float her around the pool or Jacuzzi, helping her glide through the water like a sailboat. Experiment with different motions. A rocking, cradling motion feels especially nurturing. Just make sure you keep her head up and out of the water so she doesn't get water in her eyes or nose.*

   A variation of this is to hold your partner against your body so that her head is cradled in the crook of your arm, with this same arm helping to hold up her back. This leaves your other arm free to gently caress her entire body. From time to time, gently splash water onto her torso and use it in place of massage oil to help your movements remain smooth and soothing.

❖ *During the above experience, or at another time, communicate your deepest love for your partner entirely through your hands. You can do this during a caress or massage, or whenever else you are in the mood.*

❖ *Make tender love to your partner without touching her genitals or using your own.*

❖ *Cover every inch of your partner's body with kisses.*

⑥ The Importance of Physical Affection ⑥

As discussed earlier in this book, physical affection is the glue that holds a relationship together. It is also a necessity if you plan to keep your romance alive throughout your relationship. Sadly, couples who have been together for many years often cease to be physically affectionate. Without the kissing, holding hands, hugging, and snuggling that were such clear expressions of love when they were younger, many older couples find that they have become more like roommates than lovers. If this is your situation, you can "prime the pump" by reaching out to your partner in physically demonstrative ways. When you walk past him, give him a pat on the arm or back, or better yet, the behind. When she comes home after having been out for a while, give her a welcome-home kiss, and while you're at it, make it a big wet one! In the evening, instead of just sitting in the same room together as you watch television, sit together on the couch and hold hands. Ask your partner if she would like to have her feet rubbed.

Women in particular need physical affection to become sexually interested. Many, many complain that because their husbands aren't affectionate with them, they don't really feel loved. Men also complain that since their wives aren't affectionate, they feel their wives are merely "servicing them" when they agree to have sex.

Almost As Good As Sex

Although it is true that you can continue enjoying intercourse and oral sex for as long as you wish, you may have discovered that there are other ways of connecting that feel almost as good as sex. You have nothing to prove to each other in terms of how many erections you can get or whether or not you can have an orgasm. Sometimes you just won't feel like having sex and yet you may feel a need to connect. Other times you may feel like having sex but your partner will not. Here are a few suggestions for giving each other pleasure daily, ways that may or may not stir up sexual feelings but are guaranteed to please.

1. The sensual foot caress (refer to pages 78–81 for instructions).

2. Toe stimulation. A surefire way to send pleasurable shivers all through your partner's body is to suck his or her big toe. For some, the stimulation feels so good that they describe it as a mild, continuous orgasm.

   Although sucking the big toe is particularly pleasurable, and some women love to suck the big toe as if it were a man's penis, sucking and massaging all ten toes is also delightful.

3. The Face Massage. Massaging your partner's face can release tension and can help to ease the mask we all put on to hide our feelings from the world and even from our lover.

❖ *Start by gently and lovingly holding your partner's face in your lap.*

❖ *Gently touch the outside of the ears and massage the earlobes. Many people find this especially relaxing.*

❖ *Knead the scalp and the base of the skull for further release and increased energy. Then move to the temples, which respond well to a gentle circular motion.*

❖ *Make gentle sweeping motions across the forehead using your fingers or palms.*

❖ *Starting at the chin, using the flat of both hands, gently stroke upwards alongside the jawline, the cheeks, and up to the temples. Continue the stroke up into the hair.*

❖ *Conclude by firmly but gently pressing the depression that lies at the bottom of the skull, where the head meets the neck. This will release tension in the face, head, and neck. Place a warm, wet towel over the face for a few minutes, then lift and gently dab all over the face.*

E x e r c i s e | **Discover New Erogenous Zones**

Besides the primary erogenous zone of the genitals, there are many other sensitive and highly erotic places on the body. Don't assume just because you have been together a long time that you know all your partner's likes and dislikes. Remember that our bodies and preferences change over time.

Explore all the following areas of your partner's body to discover how sensitive and erotic they feel to her or him (refer back to chapter 7 for a more detailed list):

❖ *the lips*

❖ *in and near the ears*

❖ *the nape of the neck*

❖ *the middle of the palm*

❖ *the side of the little finger*

❖ *the inner arm*

❖ *the hollows of the elbows and knees*

❖ *the nipples*

❖ *the stomach and navel*

❖ *the hollows of the buttocks*

❖ *the base of the spine*

❖ *the inner thigh*

❖ *the crease where the groin and thighs meet*

❖ *the feet*

❧ The Effects of Aging on Sexuality ❧

Although there is no such thing as being "over the hill" sexually, and no reason why older people cannot continue to enjoy sex and remain sexually active, older people do experience specific changes in sexual response as they age. When, or even if, these changes occur varies widely. Many changes may be due more to medication, chronic illness, or the psychological expectation that older people should not have sex than to the aging process itself.

During arousal, older women may experience less muscle tension, less vaginal lubrication, reduced elasticity of the vaginal walls, and little increase in breast size. The intensity of muscle spasms at orgasm may also decrease.

During arousal older men may experience the need for more time and more direct stimulation of the penis to get an erection and to reach orgasm, erections that may be less firm, and testicles that may not elevate as high up in the scrotum. At ejaculation there may be less semen, and orgasmic muscle spasms may be less intense. It is also common for men to feel less of a need to ejaculate during each sex act, and the refractory period (the time between one ejaculation and the next) may increase.

Those who don't realize that these changes are normal and that they don't necessarily decrease sexual pleasure often panic at the first sign of change. They may begin to believe that their sex lives are over, stop having sex altogether, or cease being physically affectionate with their partners.

Those who understand that these changes are normal may in fact welcome them and view this new stage in their lives as a chance to be more leisurely in their sexual encounters and less pressured by the need to perform or by the urgency for release. In fact, some couples enjoy these changes and use them to improve their sex lives. For example, men who had problems with premature ejaculation in their youth may find that the decreased urgency to ejaculate permits them to have intercourse for longer periods of time. Men who need more time to achieve an erection may now be more willing to engage in longer periods of sensual touching and intimate connecting.

Many couples who are not able to have intercourse continue to express affection and physical intimacy in other ways, such as mutual touching or oral-genital activities. As mentioned earlier, healthy and satisfying sexuality can include many different ways of physically expressing love and caring.

What most of these changes, in either women or men, require of you is more patience and fewer expectations about both you and your partner. Expecting yourself to function as you did when you were young will only add pressure to your lovemaking and might set you up for disappointment. Going slowly, opening all your senses, and focusing on the moment, as I have advocated throughout this book, will go a long way toward helping you continue to function sexually for many, many years to come. Women can maintain their sexual appetites well into their eighties and nineties. And with the advent of vascular-expanding drugs such as Viagra, even men who have been impotent for years can now achieve erections.

⑥ Illness, Surgery, and Medication ⑥

Aging is often accompanied by an increased frequency of illness, the need for surgery, and the need for medications, many of which come with certain side effects that affect sexual functioning. But you don't need to surrender your sexuality to these three inevitabilities. Unfortunately, many doctors do not prepare their patients, or their patients' partners, for the possible impact of illness, surgery, or medication on sexual functioning. Patients need to be informed about potential changes in sexual response, whether it is a lack of erection, difficulty in achieving orgasm, or diminished sex drive, so they will know what to expect and can begin to adjust to these changes.

Conversely, sometimes patients, for example, those who undergo surgery for noncancerous enlargement of the prostrate, may believe that there will be a negative effect on their erections, even though most current surgical techniques will not affect them in this way. This belief itself, however, can cause erectile problems. In other situations, men often misinterpret one change in sexual functioning (such as the absence of ejaculation at orgasm) to mean that all other functions, such as getting erections, are affected. Again, this is often not true. This is why receiving accurate information on sexual functioning is essential whenever a physician diagnoses a disease, suggests surgery, or prescribes medication.

Many older patients complain about doctors who have told them that trying for sexual functioning at their age is pointless or silly. And some doctors just seem to be embarrassed about discussing sex or refuse to discuss it at all. For these reasons, you may have to insist on a thorough explanation of how your sex life may be affected and be prepared to change physicians if you don't get satisfactory answers to your questions.

Most important, do not accept anyone's opinion that you are too old or too sick to be concerned about sex. Our increasing understanding of the immune system indicates that showing love and caring through touching and physical closeness is an important component of physical health and recovery from illness or surgery. While the road to sexual recovery isn't always smooth, those with perseverance and the patience to explore treatment options will have success in regaining sexual enjoyment. And remember, sex is not just about desire or performance, it is about pleasure and intimacy and enjoying each other as you grow older.

⑥ Loving Your Body as It Changes ⑥

Many older people are concerned about their aging bodies. They assume that their wrinkles, sagging breasts, or disappearing behinds make them less sexually attractive to their partners. It is normal for our body image to change as our bodies change.

Women who received a great deal of attention because of their physical attractiveness tend to experience the greatest difficulty making the transition from youth to maturity, since this source of automatic approval will diminish when they begin to show their age. This is especially true for women who continue to look outside themselves for approval and whose measure of their worth is based solely on their appearance.

Those women who are willing to work toward finding beauty in their aging body and toward learning to appreciate their body not only for the way it looks but for the multitude of gifts it provides will eventually grow to love and accept their bodies just as they are.

Illness, disability, and surgery can also influence the way we feel about our bodies. But staying connected to our senses can help us overcome our embarrassment and our concerns.

For example, many people, especially women, are embarrassed by surgical scars. In fact, some people are so embarrassed that it interferes with their sexuality, as was the case with Marsha. Marsha had recently had a mastectomy and was worried that Nathan, her husband of thirty-two years, would be sexually turned off by her missing breast and the scarring on her chest. I encouraged her to talk with Nathan about her concerns, and she did so. Even though he assured her that he still loved her and that he still found her attractive, she remained reluctant to let him see her naked and reported feeling completely shut down sexually.

I sensed that she needed to become more comfortable with her scars herself. I suggested that she begin by giving herself a sensual caress, rubbing oil over her entire body. Once she felt relaxed and more in touch with her body, I suggested that she spend some time caressing her surgical scar. This is what she reported: "I was very skittish about touching it at first, but when I finally did I was surprised to discover that it actually felt rather nice. It was smoother than the rest of my skin in places and I realized it wouldn't be so horrible for my husband to touch it."

But Marsha still wasn't ready to have Nathan see her scars or to touch them. I suggested she spend some time in front of the mirror, getting used to seeing herself with the missing breast. I also suggested she have her husband come in for a few sessions, and he agreed.

I spent a few minutes at the beginning of the session assuring them that their dilemma was a common one and having them express their feelings about the situation to each other. But I knew that all the talk in the world wasn't going to solve the problem. So I suggested that they engage in some of the sensate focus exercises described earlier in this book to help them take the pressure off and to reconnect with each other sensually. Marsha agreed, with the stipulation that she keep her prosthetic bra on during the exercises. They agreed and reported at subsequent sessions that the exercises had helped them both to relax and that they felt closer to each other than ever before.

The next step was to get Marsha to take her bra off and to risk Nathan's reaction. I suggested she do so in the dark at first and that she have him caress her chest with oil, as she had done herself. After Nathan reported that he enjoyed touching her scar tissue, she was finally able to allow him to caress her with the lights on.

After several more weeks of caressing exercises, Marsha reported that she felt some sexual stirrings once again and that she might be ready to resume sexual intercourse with her husband. At our last session, Marsha and Nathan were happy to report that they were once again enjoying an active sex life and that the caress exercises had helped their sex life to actually improve.

If you are concerned about such things as wrinkles, sagging muscles or breasts, or surgical scars, it is important to remember that physical attraction is mental and emotional. If someone loves you with his or her whole heart, mind, and body, it will not matter that you are missing a breast, an arm, a leg, or any other part. Continue connecting with your partner on an emotional level, sharing your deepest feelings. Continue pleasuring each other sensually and sexually. You will then find that the bond between you will continue to grow and that your partner will look at you with the light of love in his eyes, a light that shines directly to your soul.

⑥ As Long As You Keep Loving, You'll Never Grow Old ⑩

You've no doubt heard many times that a positive attitude, more than anything else, will prolong your life. The same holds true for your sex life. If you expect it to die on the vine, it no doubt will. But if you expect to remain sexually vital for the rest of your life, to continue harvesting the seeds of love you planted so long ago, you can almost guarantee that you and your partner will continue sharing exciting sensual and sexual experiences.

The following suggestions will help you to stay young at heart and in spirit.

❖ *Play a rousing game of strip poker.*

❖ *The next time you make love, say yes! out loud instead of using your usual words or sounds. In your mind you will be saying yes! to love, yes! to good health, and yes! to life.*

❖ *You've been around too long to take anything too seriously, let alone your sexual life. Make up spontaneous names for the erotic parts of your lover's body—the mouth, breasts, vagina, penis, testicles. Say them out loud:"I want to play with your pazongas." The next time you have an orgasm, try laughing to help release the tension.*

❖ *Type or write a memo to your partner that says something you want her to do that she has never done before. Start your memo with "your assignment, if you choose to accept it..." Put it in an official-looking envelope.*

❖ *Play slave/master. When you are the slave you must do everything your partner wishes. When you are the master you may ask for anything you want. (Note: this exercise may not be appropriate for survivors of rape or sexual abuse.)*

Many older people assume they will be unable to feel sensual and sexual sensations with the same intensity they once did. Or they fear that fading energy, aging bones, and weakening muscles will prevent them from engaging in the sexual activities they once enjoyed. While aging certainly slows us down, it need not put us out of commission.

All the exercises in this book will help you to remain young, vital, and sexually charged. In fact, by focusing on sensuality rather than on performance, as I have advocated throughout this book, and by continuing to connect with your senses, you will most likely find that you enjoy sex more than you did as a younger person, when sex was more forced, pressured, and goal oriented.

Some older people find that their aging skin is far more sensitive and that the sensations are intensified. Others discover that they require slightly more intense stimulation than when they were younger but that they can still feel great sexual pleasure once the pressure is deepened. Those with hearing or visual impairments will discover that their other senses, including their sense of touch, will intensify to compensate. The point is to continue to explore and experiment. With the pressures of work, raising a family, and financial concerns behind them, many older couples find that they spend far more time touching, holding, and kissing, and this in turn leads to a more active sexual life than they have experienced in years.

Finally, remember that the essence of sexuality lies in the emotional and spiritual connection we make with each other. The more you allow yourselves to open your hearts, the more your passion and sexual joy will increase. When you provide your relationship with a constant supply of love, depth, and sensuality, your lovemaking will become more and more precious and rewarding.

CONCLUSION

⑥ Sensual Sex as Time Goes By ⑥

After experiencing Sensual Sex, you will probably vow never to go back to predictable, routine sex again. Unfortunately, old habits are hard to break, and you may find your resolve fading after several months. As time goes by you may find that you once again begin to neglect your partner and your relationship. Your sensual refuge may become cluttered with the reminders of daily life, and when your bottles of essential and massage oils run out you may neglect to buy more. If any of these scenarios should come to pass, remind yourselves of why you bought this book in the first place. Remember what your relationship was like before you began the Reawakening Your Senses Program. And perhaps most important, remind each other of some of the experiences you have shared together. Refer back to your sensual journal for inspiration, to remind you of how exciting or relaxing the exercises felt, of how much intimacy you experienced together.

Just as maintaining a happy, healthy relationship requires a commitment on both your parts, continuing an exciting, passionate, and sensual relationship will require the same dedication. *Sensual Sex* can serve as a symbol of that commitment. Instead of putting this book away on a bookshelf, where it will do nothing but collect dust, leave it out on your nightstand or in your bathroom as a constant reminder to practice sensuality in your relationship and to stay connected with your senses.

Keep the commitment you made earlier to engage in some type of sensual experience together once a week, whether it be sharing a sensual body caress, taking a sensual bath together, or giving each other a foot massage after an especially difficult day. Keep up your sensual rituals and maintain your sensual refuge no matter what else is going on in your life.

The information in this book will never go out of date, no matter what new and revolutionary sexual techniques are discovered. It is my hope that you will refer to it over and over again throughout your lifetimes. Reach for it whenever you feel your relationship is suffering from boredom or neglect, whenever you question your love for your partner, or whenever you become uncertain about your partner's love. Refer to it when you feel insecure about whether your partner still finds you physically attractive or when your own feelings of attraction toward your partner begin to ebb. During times of stress, conflict, or alienation remember the intimacy you shared as you practiced some of the exercises, and allow these feelings to draw you back to each other and to the Reawakening Your Senses Program.

Refer to *Sensual Sex* for ideas whenever you wish to show your love and appreciation for your partner or whenever you want to celebrate a special occasion. Remember that all of us hunger for love, acceptance, and appreciation, and that the best way to show your partner that he is loved is to reach out with a loving touch or, better yet, a sensual massage.

There will be times when one of you wants to pursue sensuality or sex more than the other will. This is natural. When you are the more interested one, tantalize your partner with an exercise she particularly enjoyed in the past. More than likely you'll find that her sense memory will kick in and before long you'll have her eating out of the palm of your hand—literally as well as figuratively (remember the Sensuous Fruit Fest?).

When you are the less interested partner, go back through your journal or this book to find exercises that provided you with the most pleasure and that most "primed the pump," so to speak. For example, self-caressing may once again prove to be instrumental in encouraging you to engage in sensual caressing with your partner, or a sensual bath may relax you and take your mind off the pressure at work enough to get your juices flowing once again.

Most important, whenever life becomes too harried, whenever your body yearns for the healing tenderness of touch, whenever your soul craves something more meaningful and fulfilling than working or shopping, remember the power of sensuality to comfort and heal you, to fill those empty spaces inside.

Whenever your partner begins to feel more like a roommate than a lover, remember the power of Sensual Sex to connect you deeply with each other. Remember that there is more to life than facing one struggle after another. Find that meaning together by looking deeply into each other's eyes, by communicating your love through sensual touch, and by letting your tender feelings come to the surface, revealing your vulnerability and your souls.

NOTES

Chapter Three: Reconnecting with Your Five Senses

1. Valerie Gennari Cooksley, *Aromatherapy: A Lifetime Guide to Healing with Essential Oils.* (Paramus, NJ: Prentice Hall, 1996), 255.

2. This exercise was inspired by Dr. Patricia Love's book. Patricia Love and Jo Robinson, *Hot Monogamy: Essential Steps to More Passionate, Intimate Lovemaking.* (New York: Dutton, 1994), 253.

3. The Sensuous Orange exercise and the Tom Jones Dinner exercise were created by unknown sources (possibly Bernard Gunther) during the 1970s as part of the Human Potential Movement.

Chapter Four: Liquid Love

4. Cooksley, *Aromatherapy*, 12.

5. Cooksley, *Aromatherapy*, 254.

Chapter Six: Deeper Love

6. Georg Feuerstein, ed., *Sacred Sexuality: Living the Vision of the Erotic Spirit.* (New York: Tarcher/Perigee Books, 1993), 356.

7. David and Ellen Ramsdale, *Sexual Energy Ecstasy: A Practical Guide to Lovemaking Secrets of the East and West.* (New York: Bantam, 1993), xi.

Chapter Eight: Summer Love

8. Daniel Beaver, *More Than Just Sex: A Committed Couples Guide to Keeping Relationships Lively, Intimate, and Gratifying.* (Lower Lake, CA: Aslan Publishing, 1992), 78–80.

RECOMMENDED READING

Sexual Education and Enrichment

Abram, David. *The Spell of the Sensuous: Perception and Language in a More Than Human World.* New York: Vintage, 1997.

Barbach, Lonnie. *For Yourself: The Fulfillment of Female Sexuality.* Garden City, NY: Anchor Books, 1976.

―――. *For Each Other: Sharing Sexual Intimacy.* New York: New American Library, 1984.

Barbach, Lonnie and David L. Geisinger. *Going the Distance: Finding and Keeping Lifelong Love.* New York: New American Library, 1993.

Engel, Beverly. *Raising Your Sexual Self-Esteem.* New York: Fawcett Columbine, 1995.

Henderson, Julie. *The Lover Within: Opening to Energy in Sexual Practice.* Barrytown, NY: Station Hill Press, 1987.

Hirsch, Alan R. *Scentsational Sex: The Secret to Using Aroma for Arousal.* Boston: Element Books, 1998.

Kitzinger, Sheila. *Woman's Experience of Sex: The Facts and Feelings of Female Sexuality at Every Stage of Life.* New York: Penguin Books, 1993.

Montague, Ashley. *Touching: The Human Significance of the Skin.* New York: Harper & Row, 1986.

Zilbergeld, Bernie. *Male Sexuality: A Guide to Sexual Fulfillment.* Boston: Little, Brown, 1978.

Intimacy and Relationship Enhancement

Beaver, Daniel. *More Than Just Sex: A Committed Couples Guide to Keeping Relationships Lively, Intimate, and Gratifying.* Lower Lake, CA: Aslan Publishing, 1992.

Covington, Stephanie. *Leaving the Enchanted Forest: The Path from Relationship Addiction to Intimacy.* San Francisco: Harper & Row, 1988.

Hendrix, Harville. *Getting the Love You Want.* New York: Harper & Row, 1988.

Lerner, Harriet. *The Dance of Intimacy: A Woman's Guide to Courageous Acts of Change in Key Relationships.* New York: Harper & Row, 1989.

Love, Patricia and Jo Robinson. *Hot Monogamy: Essential Steps to More Passionate, Intimate Lovemaking.* New York: Dutton, 1994.

Maltz, Wendy. *Passionate Hearts: The Poetry of Sexual Love*. San Rafael, CA: New World Library, 1996.

Moore, Thomas. *Soul Mates*. New York: HarperCollins, 1994.

Scarf, Maggie. *Intimate Partners: Patterns in Love and Marriage*. New York: Random House, 1978.

Woititz, Janet. *Struggle for Intimacy*. Pompano Beach, FL.: Health Communications, 1985.

Massage

Rush, Anne Kent. *A Romantic Massage: Ten Unforgettable Massages for Special Occasions*. New York: Avon, 1991.

Essential Oils and Aromatherapy

Cooksley, Valerie Gennari. *Aromatherapy: A Lifetime Guide to Healing with Essential Oils*. Paramus, NJ: Prentice Hall, 1996.

Watson, Cynthia. *Love Potions*. Los Angeles: Tarcher, 1993.

Sacred Sexuality

Anand, Margo. *The Art of Sexual Ecstasy*. Los Angeles: Tarcher, 1989.

Feuerstein, Georg, ed. *Enlightened Sexuality*. Freedom, CA: The Crossing Press, 1989.

————. *Sacred Sexuality: Living the Vision of the Erotic Spirit*. New York: Tarcher/Perigee Books, 1993.

Garrison, Omar. *Tantra: The Yoga of Sex*. New York: Avon Books, 1973.

Moffett, Robert. *Tantric Sex*. New York: Berkley Medallion, 1974.

Muir, Charles and Caroline. *Tantra: The Art of Conscious Loving*. San Francisco: Mercury House, 1989.

Ramsdale, David and Ellen. *Sexual Energy Ecstasy: A Practical Guide to Lovemaking Secrets of the East and West*. New York: Bantam, 1993.

Rituals, Spiritual Journal Writing, Prayers

Baldwin, Christina. *Life's Companion: Journal Writing as a Spiritual Quest*. New York: Bantam, 1990.

Imber-Black, Evan and Janine Roberts. *Rituals for Our Times*. New York: HarperCollins, 1992.

Steindl-Rast, Brother David. *Gratefulness: The Heart of Prayer*. New York: Paulist Press, 1984.

Erotica

Alvrez, Alicia. *On The Wings of Eros: Nightly Readings for Passion and Romance.* Berkeley, CA: Conari Press, 1995.

Chester, Laura. *The Unmade Bed.* New York: HarperCollins, 1992.

Your Body and Body Image

The Boston Women's Health Book Collective. *The New Our Bodies, Ourselves.* New York: Simon & Schuster, 1984. (A complete sourcebook on women's healthcare issues, from birthing to aging.)

Chernin, Kim. *The Obsession: Reflections on the Tyranny of Slenderness.* New York: Harper & Row, 1981.

Hutchinson, Marcia Germaine. *Transforming Body Image.* Freedom, CA: Crossing Press, 1988. (Step-by-step exercises to help integrate your body, mind, and self-image and to begin loving and accepting yourself just the way you are.)

McFarland, Barbara and Tyeis Baker-Baumann. *Shame and Body Image: Culture and the Compulsive Eater.* Deerfield Beach, FL.: Health Communications, 1990.

Sex and Aging

Barbach, Lonnie. *The Pause: Positive Approaches to Menopause.* New York: Signet, 1994.

Burnett, R. G. *Menopause: All Your Questions Answered.* Chicago: Contempory Books, Inc., 1987.

Butler, R. N. and M. I. Lewis. *Love and Sex After 60.* New York: Harper & Row, 1988.

Cutler, W. B., C.R. Garcia, and D. A. Edwards. *Menopause: A Guide for Women and the Men Who Love Them.* New York: Norton, 1983.

Doress, P. B. et al. *Ourselves, Growing Older: Women Aging with Knowledge and Power.* New York: Simon and Schuster, 1987.

Schover, L. R. *Prime Time: Sexual Health for Men Over Fifty.* New York: Holt, Rinehart and Winston, 1984.

Illness, Surgery, Disabilities, and Sex

Cutler, W. B. *Hysterectomy: Before and After.* New York: Harper & Row, 1988.

Schover, R. and S. B. Jensen. *Sexuality and Chronic Illness: A Comprehensive Approach.* New York: The Guilford Press, 1988.

Weiner, Florence. *No Apologies: A Guide to Living with a Disability.* New York: St. Martin's Press, 1986.

Sexual Dysfunction

Heiman, Julia and Joseph LoPiccolo. *Becoming Orgasmic: A Sexual and Personal Growth Program for Women.* New York: Prentice Hall, 1988.

Kaplan, Helen Singer. *The New Sex Therapy: Active Treatment of Sexual Dysfunctions.* New York: Brunner/Mazel, 1974.

————. *How to Overcome Premature Ejaculation.* New York: Brunner/Mazel, 1989.

Keesling, Barbara. *Sexual Healing: A Self-Help Program to Enhance Your Sensuality and Overcome Common Sexual Problems.* Alameda, CA: Hunter House, 1990.

Knoph, Jennifer and Michael Sieler. *I.S.D.: Inhibited Sexual Desire.* New York: William Morrow, 1990.

Masters, William and Virginia Johnson. *Human Sexual Inadequacy.* Boston: Little, Brown, 1970.

Childhood Sexual Abuse

RECOVERY

Bass, Ellen and Laura Davis. *The Courage to Heal: A Guide for Women Survivors of Child Sexual Abuse.* New York: Harper & Row, 1988. Includes a section on intimacy and sexuality.

Engel, Beverly. *The Right to Innocence: Healing the Trauma of Childhood Sexual Abuse.* New York: Ballantine, 1991.

Lew, Mike. *Victims No Longer: Men Recovering from Incest and Other Sexual Child Abuse.* New York: HarperCollins, 1990. Includes general information about the sexual effects of abuse on sexuality; also includes a helpful section on dealing with confusion about sexual orientation.

SEXUAL RECOVERY

Maltz, Wendy and Beverly Holman. *Incest and Sexuality: A Guide to Understanding and Healing.* San Francisco: Jossey Bass, 1993.

Maltz, Wendy. *The Sexual Healing Journey: A Guide for Survivors of Sexual Abuse.* New York: HarperPerennial, 1992.

HELP FOR PARTNERS OF RAPE AND CHILD SEXUAL ABUSE

Engel, Beverly. *Partners in Recovery: How Mates, Lovers & Other Prosurvivors Can Learn to Cope with Adult Survivors of Childhood Sexual Abuse.* New York: Fawcett Columbine, 1991.

McEnvoy, Alan and Jeff Brookings. *If She Is Raped: A Book for Husbands, Fathers, and Male Friends.* Holmes Beach, FL: Learning Publications, 1984.

Schneider, Jennifer. *Back from Betrayal: Surviving His Affairs.* New York: Harper & Row, 1988.

Safe Sex

Institute for Advanced Study of Human Sexuality. *The Complete Guide to Safer Sex.* Fort Lee, NJ: Barricade, 1992.

Homosexuality and Bisexuality

Berzon, Betty. *Positively Gay.* Los Angeles: Mediamix Associates, 1979.

Bode, Janet. *View from Another Closet: Exploring Bisexuality in Women.* New York: Pocket Books, 1977.

Loulan, J. *Lesbian Sex.* San Francisco: Spinster's Ink., 1984. Written by a lesbian counselor in a nontechnical style. Features sections on sex and disability, sobriety, sexual abuse, and aging.

————. *Lesbian Passion: Loving Ourselves and Each Other.* San Francisco: Spinsters/Aunt Lute, 1987. Addresses self-esteem, intimacy, and relationship issues.

McWhirter, D. P. and A. M. Mattison. *The Male Couple: How Relationships Develop.* Englewood Cliffs, NJ: Prentice-Hall, 1984.

RESOURCES

Essential Oils

Aroma Vera
3384 S. Robertson Pl.
Los Angeles, CA 90034
In California: (310) 280-0407
Outside California: (800) 669-9514

Herb Products Co.
11012 Magnolia Blvd.
North Hollywood, CA 91601
(818) 984-3141

Erotica, Massage Oils, and Vibrators

Eve's Garden
119 West 57th St., Ste. 420
New York, NY 10019
Their goal is to "offer women the space
to enjoy, expand, and celebrate their
sexuality." Write for catalog.

Good Vibrations
1219 Valencia St.
San Francisco, CA 94110
Call for catalogs: (415) 974-8990

It's My Pleasure
4526 S.E. Hawthorne
Portland, OR 97215
(503) 236-0505

Sensuality and Personal Growth Seminars

Esalen Institute
Big Sur, CA 93920
Catalog requests: (408) 644-8476

Grof Transpersonal Training
Holotropic Breath Work
20 Sunnyside Ave., Ste. A-314
Mill Valley, CA 94941

Sacred Sexuality Seminars

Sexual Energy Ecstasy Seminars
Box 5489
Playa Del Rey, CA 90296

Kahua Institute
Box 1747
Makawao, Maui, HI 96768

Source Retreats
Box 69
Paia, Maui, HI 96779.

Deer Tribe
Box 1519
Temple City, CA 91780.

Tantric Videos

Intimacy and Sexual Ecstasy
Love Alive Productions
Box 1045
Santa Barbara, CA 93102

Tantra Love
Skill Publishing
Box 5489
Playa Del Rey, CA 90296

Organizations

Society for the Scientific Study of Sex
Box 208
Mount Vernon, IA 52314

National Sex Forum
1523 Franklin St.
San Francisco, CA 94109

American Holistic Medical Association
6932 Little River Turnpike
Annandale, VA 22003

AIDS Hotline of U.S. Public Health
Service
(800) 922-AIDS
Tape: (800) 342-AIDS

How to Locate a Sex Therapist or Marriage Counselor

❖ If you are comfortable doing so, ask friends, family members, or coworkers who have gone to a counselor whether they can recommend someone.

❖ Ask your family physician or clergy-man for a recommendation.

❖ Write to one of the following groups and ask for a list of certified counselors and therapists in your area (there may be a nominal fee):

American Association of Sex Educators, Counselors and Therapists (AASECT)
11 Dupont Circle N.W., Ste. 220
Washington, DC 20036

American Association for Marriage and Family Therapy (AAMFT)
1717 K. St. N.W., Ste. 407
Washington, DC 20006

For Sexual Dysfunction:

❖ Call your local community health center and ask for recommenda-tions, or call the nearest medical school or large hospital and ask if they have a sex dysfunction clinic.

❖ Call the nearest medical school, uni-versity, or large hospital and ask if they have a special clinic for diag-nosing and treating sexual problems (dysfunctions). If your town does not have such a facility, most libraries have telephone directories of nearby large cities.

❖ Look in the yellow pages of your
  telephone book under:

  Marriage, Family, Child
  Counselors

  Psychologists

  Psychiatrists (may be listed
  under Physicians or Surgeons)

  Mental Health Services

If you suspect your sexual or relationship problems may include medical or
physical factors, locate a sex therapist
who works closely with medical profes-
sionals or a physician with special training in sexual medicine.

Help for Survivors of Childhood Sexual Abuse or Rape

VOICES (Victims of Incest Can Emerge
Survivors) in Action, Inc.
P.O. Box 148309
Chicago, IL 60614
(312) 327-1500

A national network of female and male
survivors and prosurvivors that has
local groups and contacts throughout
the country. Offers a free referral service that provides listings of therapists,
agencies, and self-help groups.

Incest Survivors Anonymous (ISA)
P.O. Box 5613
Long Beach, CA 90805
(213) 428-5599

Survivors of Incest Anonymous
World Service Office
P.O. Box 21817
Baltimore, MD 21222
(301) 282-3400

Videos:

"Relearning Touch: Healing Techniques
for Couples" and "Partners in Healing:
Couples Overcoming the Sexual
Repercussions of Incest." (Created by
Wendy Maltz)

Independent Video Services
401 E. 10th Ave., Ste. 160
Eugene, OR 97401
(800) 678-3455

INDEX

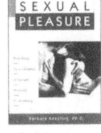
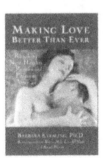

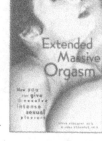
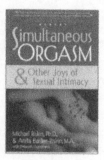

A PORTABLE SEXUALITY LIBRARY
Four Pocketbooks *by* Richard Craze

THE POCKET BOOK OF SENSATIONAL ORGASMS

Designed for couples in loving relationships, this is a unique look at how couples can intensify, extend, and enhance orgasms.

Using techniques such as "The Tail of the Ostrich" and the "Two-Handed-Twist," partners can release inhibitions and can share erotic adventures. The book also explains the difference between male and female orgasms; types of orgasms: vaginal, clitoral, G-Spot, anal, multiple, mutual, and oral; and how to magnify sexual satisfaction with seduction and foreplay.

96 pages ... 64 color photos ... Paperback $11.95 ... OCTOBER 2002

THE POCKET BOOK OF FOREPLAY

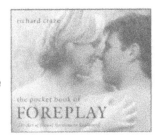

Foreplay isn't just a prelude to the "real thing"—it's an experience to be enjoyed for itself. This book shows you how, with full-color pictures of the joys of foreplay, from "Setting the Scene" to "Reaching the Limits" it's full of new foreplay ideas and even sexy Tantric techniques.

96 pages ... 68 color photos ... Paperback $10.95

THE POCKET BOOK OF SEX AND CHOCOLATE

What more could a body want? Explore the pleasures of the ultimate combination—sex and chocolate. The suggestions in this book for combining chocolate and sex range from saucy to classy. You learn about the best kinds of chocolate—and how to smear, lick, dribble, and, of course, eat it. Full of sensuous photographs, this book will give new meaning to the joy of chocolate.

96 pages ... 67 color photos ... Paperback $10.95

THE POCKET BOOK OF SEXUAL FANTASIES

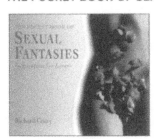

Our imagination knows no bounds when it comes to sex and passion. This book explores how to get beyond inhibitions and act out fantasies. It guides you through the common kinds of fantasy—bondage, striptease, voyeurism, fetishism, toys, teasing, leather and lace, exhibitionism, and cross-dressing—and touches on how fantasy can become an art form or even a ritual.

96 pages ... 64 color photos ... Paperback $10.95

To order or for our FREE catalog or call (800) 266-5592

Printed in the USA
CPSIA information can be obtained
at www.ICGtesting.com
JSHW082158140824
68134JS00014B/301

9 780897 932455